The Reproductive System at a Glance

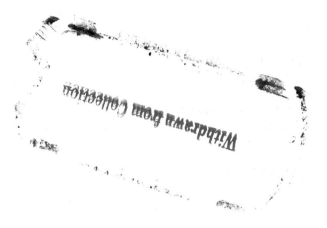

The Reproductive System at a Glance

Linda J. Heffner

MD, PhD
Professor and Chair
Department of Obstetrics and Gynecology
Boston University School of Medicine
Chief of Obstetrics and Gynecology
Boston Medical Center
Boston
USA

Danny J. Schust

MD
Associate Professor of Obstetrics and Gynecology
Division of Reproductive Biology
Department of Obstetrics and Gynecology
Boston Medical Center
Boston University School of Medicine
Boston
USA

Second Edition

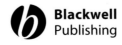
Blackwell
Publishing

© 2006 Linda J. Heffner, Danny J. Schust
Published by Blackwell Publishing Ltd
Blackwell Publishing, Inc., 350 Main Street, Malden, Massachusetts 02148-5020, USA

Blackwell Publishing Ltd, 9600 Garsington Road, Oxford OX4 2DQ, UK
Blackwell Publishing Asia Pty Ltd, 550 Swanston Street, Carlton, Victoria 3053, Australia

First published 2001
Second Edition 2006
3   2008

Library of Congress Cataloging-in-Publication Data

Heffner, Linda J.
    The reproductive system at a glance/Linda J. Heffner, Danny J. Schust.—2nd ed.
        p.; cm. — (At a glance)
    Rev. ed. of: Human reproduction at a glance/Linda J. Heffner. 2001.
    Includes index.
    ISBN 978-1-4051-2983-1 (alk. paper)
    1. Human reproduction.   2. Reproductive health.   3. Generative organs—Diseases.
    [DNLM: 1. Reproduction—physiology.   2. Genital Diseases, Female.   3. Genital Diseases, Male.
    4. Pregnancy Complications.   5. Sexually Transmitted Diseases. WQ 205 H461p 2005]
    I. Schust, Danny J.   II. Heffner, Linda J. Human reproduction at a glance.   III. Title.
    IV. Series: At a glance series (Oxford, England)

QP251.H39 2005
612.6—dc22

                                                                                2005017261

ISBN 978-1-4051-2983-1

A catalogue record for this title is available from the British Library

Set in 9/11.5 Times by Graphicraft Limited, Hong Kong
Printed and bound in Malaysia by Vivar Printing Sdn. Bhd.

Commissioning Editor: Martin Sugden
Editorial Assistant: Caroline Adders
Development Editor: Mirjana Misina
Production Controller: Kate Charman

For further information on Blackwell Publishing, visit our website: http://www.blackwellpublishing.com

Contents

Preface

The Reproductive System at a Glance, while it has a new title, is actually the second edition of a textbook that I wrote five years ago in an attempt to collate all the pertinent information on human reproductive processes and their diseases into one easy-to-use overview. It is intended as both a learning and study guide for medical students and physicians who wish to have a comprehensive overview of the anatomy, physiology and pathophysiology of the reproductive systems in men and women.

This new edition has been substantially revised both to update the retained material and to replace less useful sections with more relevant materials. Most notably, chapters on placental structure and function, genetic imprinting and reproductive tract cancers, and HIV infection have replaced the two overview chapters (common mechanisms in endocrine disorders and the overview of neoplasia) and the chapter on hirsutism and androgenic alopecia. Dr. Danny Schust, my capable new co-author, has spearheaded a complete re-editing of all the original text as well as organizing the new material. The net result, we believe, is an up-to-date, comprehensive and exceptionally clear text.

For ease of use, the book remains divided into two parts. Part I, which consists of 25 chapters, covers normal human reproduction beginning with the embryology of the reproductive tract, through puberty with the resulting mature male and female anatomy and physiology and on to procreation, pregnancy and menopause. Part II, which consists of 22 chapters, covers the pathophysiology of anatomical, physiological and psychological disorders that interfere with normal reproductive function or health. Seven of these chapters are devoted to the more common malignancies that involve the reproductive organs.

Like its predecessor and the other books in this series, *The Reproductive System at a Glance* is written so that each topic is confined to a discrete vignette with appropriate illustrations or tables in a facing page format. In Part II, each topic also follows a standard format of a description of the disorder followed by its epidemiology, pathophysiology and, whenever it aids in understanding the disorder, a brief description of the commonly used treatments.

Revising a book, while easier than writing the original, remains a major undertaking to which many people contributed. I would like to thank Dr. Schust for his energy and enthusiasm in taking on the task of editing the original material and writing much of the new. Catrina McMahan, his assistant, drew some amazing new computer-based diagrams to accompany the new material we sent to Blackwell Science. Second year medical students at Boston University School of Medicine made many helpful comments after using the book for the first time.

Finally, books never appear in print or on bookshelves with publishers. I would like to thank Mirjana Misina, Richard Spilsbury and Martin Sugden at Blackwell Publishing for their assistance in producing this new edition. David Gardner, their professional illustrator, was invaluable in drawing and revising both the new and old figures.

Linda J. Heffner
Boston, 2005

Table & Figure Acknowledgements

The following figures (page numbers in roman) and tables (page numbers in italics) have been redrawn from the originals and were used with permission of the publishers. Every effort has been made by the authors to contact all copyright holders to obtain their permission to reproduce copyright material. However, if any have been inadvertently overlooked, the publisher will be pleased to make the necessary arrangements at the earliest opportunity.

2 Gonadotropins
p.12: Braunstein G (1989) Placental hormones, hormonal preparation for and control of parturition, and hormonal diagnosis of pregnancy. In: *Endocrinology* (ed. LJ deGroot), p.2045. Elsevier, Philadelphia.
And
Halvorsen LM, Chin WW (1999) Gonadotropic hormones: biosynthesis, secretion, receptors, and action. In: *Reproductive Endocrinology* (eds SSC Yen, RB Jaffe, RL Barbieri), p.92. Elsevier, Philadelphia.

3 Steroid hormones
p.14: Dr Susan Haas, Boston University School of Medicine, Boston Medical Center, Boston.
p.15: Yeh J, Adashi EY (1999) The ovarian life cycle. In: *Reproductive Endocrinology* (eds SSC Yen, RB Jaffe, RL Barbieri), p.168. Elsevier, Philadelphia.

4 Steroid hormone mechanism of action and metabolism
p.16: O'Malley BW, Strott CA (1999) Steroid hormones: metabolism and mechanism of action. In: *Reproductive Endocrinology* (eds SSC Yen, RB Jaffe, RL Barbieri), p.124. Elsevier, Philadelphia.

5 Reproductive genetics
p.18: Morton CC, Miron P (1999) Cytogenetics. In: *Reproduction in Reproductive Endocrinology* (eds SSC Yen, RB Jaffe, RL Barbieri), p.337. Elsevier, Philadelphia.
p.19: Johnson MH, Everitt BJ (1995) *Essential Reproduction*, p.2. Blackwell Science, Oxford.

6 Gonadal development in the embryo
p.20: adapted from: Morton CC, Miron P (1999) Cytogenetics. In: *Reproduction in Reproductive Endocrinology* (eds SSC Yen, RB Jaffe, RL Barbieri), p.337. Elsevier, Philadelphia.
p.21: Williams PL, Wendell-Smith CP, Treadgold S (1966) *Basic Human Embryology*, p.76. Lippincott Williams & Wilkins, Baltimore.

7 Phenotypic sex differentiation
p.22: Blainsky BI (1970) *An Introduction to Embryology*, 3rd edn, p.497. Elsevier, Philadelphia.
p.23: Williams PL, Wendell-Smith CP, Treadgold S (1966) *Basic Human Embryology*, p.78. Lippincott Williams & Wilkins, Baltimore.

8 Gross anatomy of the male reproductive tract
p.24: Romanes GJ (1972) *Cunninghams's Textbook of Anatomy*, 11th edn, pp.525, 531, 533. Oxford University Press, Oxford

9 Microscopic anatomy of the male reproductive tract
p.26, left: Bloom W, Fawcett DW (1969) *A Textbook of Histology*, 9th edn, p.688. Dr Don W Fawcett, Montana.
p.26, right: Clermont Y (1972) Kinetics of spermatogenesis in mammals: seminiferous epithelium cycle and spermatogonial renewal. *Physiol Rev* **52**: 206

10 Gross anatomy of the female reproductive tract
p.28: Netter FH (1954) *The Ciba Collection of Medical Illustrations: Vol 2, The Reproductive System*, p.110. Ciba, New Jersey.
p.29: Romanes GJ (1972) *Cunningham's Textbook of Anatomy*, 11th edn, p.544 Oxford University Press, Oxford.

11 Microscopic anatomy of the female reproductive tract.
p.30: Turner CD (1966) *General Endocrinology*, 5th edn, p.400. Elsevier, Philadelphia.
p.31: Netter FH (1954) *The Ciba Collection of Medical Illustrations: Vol 2, The Reproductive System*, pp.115, 118–9. Ciba, New Jersey.

12 Puberty in boys
p.32: Marshall WA, Tanner JM (1970) Variations in pattern of pubertal changes in boys. *Arch Dis Child* **45**: 13–23.

13 Puberty in girls
p.34: Marshall, WA, Tanner JM (1969) Variations in pattern of pubertal changes in girl. *Arch Dis Child* **44**: 291–301.

14 Male reproductive physiology
p.36 (a): Jordan GH (1999) Erectile function and dysfunction. *Postgrad Med* **105**: 133.
p.36 (b): Guiliano FA, Rampin O, Benoit G, Jardin A (1995) Neural control of penile erection. *Urol Clin North Am* **22**: 748.

15 The menstrual cycle
p.38: Groome, NP, Illingworth PJ, O'Brien M *et al.* (1996) Measurement of dimeric inhibin B throughout the human menstrual cycle. *J Clin Endocrinol Metab* **81**: 1401–5.
And
Marshall JC, Odell WD. (1989) The menstrual cycle-hormonal regulation, mechanisms of anovulation and responses of the reproductive tract to steroid hormones. In: *Endocrinology* (ed. L DeGroot), p.1946. Elsevier, Philadelphia.

16 Human sexual response
p.40: Masters WH, Johnson VE (1966) *Human Sexual Response*, p.5. Lippincott Williams & Wilkins, Baltimore.

17 Fertilization and the establishment of pregnancy
p.42 Alberts B, Bray D, Lewis J *et al.* (1994) *Molecular Biology of the Cell*, p.1031. Garland Science/ Taylor and Francis, New York.

19 The protein hormones of pregnancy
p.46: Yen SSC (1989) Endocrinology of pregnancy. In: *Maternal–Fetal Medicine* (eds RK Creasy, R Resnik), 2nd edn, p.385. Elsevier, Philadelphia.

p.47: Jaffe RB, (1999) Neuroendocrine-metabolic regulation of pregnancy. In: *Reproductive Endocrinology* (eds SSC Yen, RB Jaffe, RL Barbieri), p.767. Elsevier, Philadelphia.
And
Liu JH, Rebar RW (1999) Endocrinology of pregnancy. In: *Maternal–Fetal Medicine* (eds RK Creasy, R Resnik), 2nd edn, p.386. Elsevier, Philadelphia.

20 The steroid hormones of pregnancy
p.48: Friesen HG, Cowden EA (1989) Lactation and galactorrhea. In: *Endocrinology* (ed. LJ deGroot), 2nd edn, p.2076. Elsevier, Philadelphia.
p.49: Yen SSC (1989) Endocrinology of pregnancy. In: *Maternal–Fetal Medicine* (eds RK Creasy, R Resnik), 2nd edn, p.377, 380, 382. Elsevier, Philadelphia.

22 Labour
pp.52, 53: Challis JGR, Gibb W (1996) Control of parturition. *Prenat Neonat Med* **1**: 284.

23 The breast and lactation
p.54, left: Lyons WP (1958) Hormonal synergism in mammary growth. *Proc R Soc Lond B* **149**: 303.
p.55, right: Worthington-Roberts BS (1997) Lactation: basic considerations. In: *Nutrition in Pregnancy and Lactation* (eds BS Worthington-Roberts, SR Williams), 6th edn, p.320. McGraw-Hill, New York.

26 Abnormalities of male sexual differentiation and development
p.60: Williams PL, Wendell-Smith CP, Treadgold S (1996) *Basic Human Embryology*, p.81. Lippincott Williams & Wilkins, Baltimore.
p.61: Griffin JE. (1992) Androgen resistance- the clinical and molecular spectrum. *N Eng J Med* **326**: 612.

27 Abnormalitites of female sexual differentialtion and development.
p.62: Williams, PL, Wendell-Smith CP, Treadgold S (1966) *Basic Human Embryology*, p.81. Lippincott Williams & Wilkins, Baltimore.

28 Precocious puberty
pp.64, 65: Miller WL, Styne DM (1999) Female puberty and its disorders. In: *Reproductive Endocrinology* (eds SCC Yen, RB Jaffe, RL Barbieri), pp.394, 397. Elsevier, Philadelphia.

29 Delayed puberty
p.67: Miller WL, Styne DM (1999) Female puberty and its disorders. In: *Reproductive Endocrinology* (eds SCC Yen, RB Jaffe, RL Barbieri), p.401. Elsevier, Philadelphia.

30 Primary amenorrhoea
p.68: Barbieri RL (1997) Approach to menstrual disorders and galactorrhea. In: *Textbook of Internal Medicine* (ed. WN Kelley), 3rd edn, p.2146. Lippincott Williams & Wilkins, Baltimore.

31 Secondary amenorrhoea
p.70: Barbieri RL (1997) Approach to menstrual disorders and galactorrhea. In: *Textbook of Internal Medicine* (ed. WN Kelley), 3rd edn, p.2147. Lippincott Williams & Wilkins, Baltimore.

32 Hyperprolactinaemia
p.72: Yen SCC, Jaffe RB (1999) Prolactin in human reproduction In: *Reproductive Endocrinology* (eds SCC Yen, RB Jaffe, RL Barbieri), p.261. Elsevier, Philadelphia.

33 Sexual dysfunction
p.74: Kaplan HS (1995) *The Sexual Desire Disorders*, p.17. Brunner/ Routledge, Taylor and Francis Publishing, New York.

35 Multifetal pregnancy
p.78: FitzGerald MJT, FitzGerald M (1994) *Human Embryology*, p.51. Ballière Tindall/ Elsevier, Philadelphia.

36 Spontaneous pregnancy loss
p.79: Adapted from: Huszar G (1989) Physiology of the myometrium. In: *Maternal–Fetal Medicine* (eds R Creasy, R Resnik), 2nd edn, p.147. Elsevier, Philadelphia.
p.79: Thompson MW (1986) *Thompson and Thompson's Genetics in Medicine*, 4th edn. Elsevier, Philadelphia.

38 Breast cancer
p.84: Lopez-Otin C, Diamondis EP (1998) Breast and prostate cancer: an analysis of common epidemiological, genetic, and biochemical features. *Endocr Rev* **19**: 383.
p.85: Marchant DJ (1997) *Risk factors in breast disease* (ed. DJ Marchant), pp.116, 119. Elsevier, Philadelphia.

39 Testicular tumours
p.86: Walt H *et al.* (1992) Characterization of precancerous and neoplastic human testicular germ cells. In: *Pathobiology of Human Germ Cell Neoplasia* (eds JW Osterhuis, H Walt, I Damjanov). *Rec Results Can Res* **123**: 41.

40 Diseases of the prostate
p.88, left: Kirby R, Christmas T (1993) *Anatomy, Embryology and Histopathology in Benign Prostatic Hypertrophy*, p.18. Elsevier, Philadelphia.
p. 88, right: Lepor H, Lawson RK, (1993) *Prostate Diseases*, p.45. Elsevier, Philadelphia.

41 Ovarian neoplasms
p.91: DiSaia PJ, Creasman RK (1997) Epithelial ovarian cancer. In: *Clinical Gynecologic Oncology*, 5th edn, p.283. Elsevier, Philadelphia.

42 Endometrial cancer
p.93: Mencaglia L, Tonellotto D, Tiso E (1999) Epidemiology of endometrial carcinoma. In: *Endometrial Carcinoma and its Precursors* (eds L. Mencagaia, RF Valle, Lurain), p.2. Isis Medical Media/Taylor and Francis, New York. Adapted from Armstrong BK, Doll R (1975) Environmental factors and cancer incidence and motrtality in difference countries with special reference to dietary practices. *Int J Cancer* **15**: 617.

43 Cervical cancer
p.94: Coleman DV, Evans DMD (1998) *Biopsy Pathology and Cytology of the Cervix*. CRC Press/Taylor and Francis, New York

p.95: Walboomers JMM, de Roda Husman A-M, van den Brule AJC, Snijders PJF, Meijer CJLM (1994) Detection of genital human papillomavirus infections: critical review of methods and prevalence studies in relation to cervical cancer. In: *Human Papillomaviruses and Cervical Cancer* (eds PL Stern, MA Stanley), p.61. Oxford University Press, Oxford.

44 Genetic imprinting and reproductive tract tumours

p.96: Szulman AE, Surti U (1984) The syndromes of partial and complete molar gestation. *Clin Obstet Gynecol* **27**: 177.

45 Sexually transmitted diseases of bacterial origin

p.98: Diallabetta G, Hook EW, III (1987) Gonococcal infections. *Infect Dis Clin N Amer* **1**: 1,28.

p.99: Batteiger BE, Jones RB (1987) Chlamydial infections. *Infect Dis Clin N Amer* **1**: 1,58.

46 Sexually transmitted diseases of viral origin

p.101: Arrand JR, (1994) Molecular genetics of human papillomaviruses. In: *Human Papillomaviruses and Cervical Cancer* (eds PL Stern, MA Stanley), pp.28–40. Oxford University Press, Oxford.

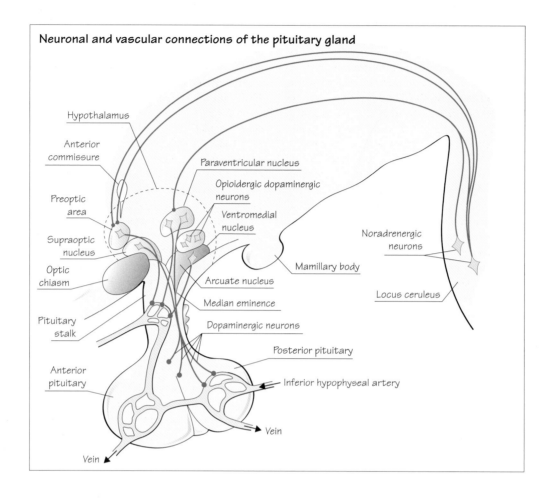

Neuronal and vascular connections of the pituitary gland

Hypothalamus

Anterior commissure

Preoptic area

Supraoptic nucleus

Optic chiasm

Pituitary stalk

Anterior pituitary

Vein

Paraventricular nucleus

Opioidergic dopaminergic neurons

Ventromedial nucleus

Arcuate nucleus

Median eminence

Dopaminergic neurons

Mamillary body

Noradrenergic neurons

Locus ceruleus

Posterior pituitary

Inferior hypophyseal artery

Vein

Structure and function

There are three lobes to the pituitary gland (hypophysis). The **anterior lobe** (adenohypophysis) is derived embryologically from ectoderm lining the dorsal pharynx, which forms an outpocketing known as Rathke's pouch. The **posterior lobe** (neurohypophysis) is much smaller and derived embryologically from neuroectoderm. The **pars intermedia**, a small intermediate structure lying between the anterior and posterior lobes, is actually a subdivision of the anterior lobe. Importantly, the embryological anlage of the pituitary gland is derived from neural crest cells.

The pituitary is connected to the brain via a small stalk of tissue known as the pituitary stalk or infundibulum. The posterior pituitary serves mainly as a storage site. Two hormones are stored here: oxytocin and arginine vasopressin (also known as antidiuretic hormone, ADH). Both are produced in the hypothalamus. Axons from large cell (magnocellular) neurons in the anterior hypothalamus travel into the posterior pituitary through the posterior part of the infundibulum. The oxytocin and ADH synthesized in the neuronal cell bodies of these hypothalamic cells travel down their axons, where the two hormones are then stored in the posterior pituitary. In contrast, the anterior pituitary produces its own tropic hormones under the regulatory control of the hypothalamus. This control is mediated by neuroendocrine signals from the hypothalamus that travel through rich vascular connections surrounding the pituitary stalk. Axons from small cell (parvocellular) neurons in the

hypothalamus end in the precapillary space of the primary portal system that originates at the base of the hypothalamus. Blood flowing through this highly vascular plexus delivers signals to the anterior pituitary gland, regulating production and release of its protein products.

There are five small cell types in the anterior pituitary that are associated with tropic hormone production: gonadotropes, lactotropes, somatotropes, thyrotropes and corticotropes. These specific cells are responsible for production and secretion of: **follicle-stimulating hormone (FSH)** and **luteinizing hormone (LH)**; **prolactin**; **growth hormone**; **thyroid-stimulating hormone (TSH)**; and **adrenocorticotropic hormone (ACTH)**, respectively. The thyrotropes and gonadotropes closely resemble each other histologically because their secretory products, LH, FSH and TSH, are all glycoprotein hormones (Chapter 2) that stain with carbohydrate-sensitive reagents. LH and FSH are produced by a single cell type, allowing coupled secretion and regulation by a single releasing factor.

Control of the activity of the pituitary gland comes largely from the hypothalamus with important direct modulation by feedback mechanisms. The hypothalamic nuclei associated with reproduction include the supraoptic, paraventricular, arcuate, ventromedial and suprachiasmatic nuclei. Neurons in two less well-defined areas, the medial anterior hypothalamus and the medial preoptic areas, are also involved. The magnocellular (large) neurons that originate in the supraoptic and paraventricular nuclei project into the posterior pituitary and produce the hormones vasopressin and oxytocin. The parvocellular (small) neurons are found in the paraventricular, arcuate and ventromedial nuclei and the periventricular and medial preoptic areas. The parvocellular neurons produce regulatory peptides that control gonadotrope, lactotrope, somatotrope, thyrotrope and corticotrope cell function.

Those cells in the hypothalamic nuclei that regulate the pituitary have several functions. They receive signals from higher centres in the brain, they generate neural signals of their own and they have neuroendocrine capabilities. The higher areas of the brain that connect to the hypothalamic nuclei involved with reproduction are the locus ceruleus, the medulla and pons, the midbrain raphe, the olfactory bulb, the limbic system (amygdala and hippocampus), the piriform cortex and the retina. Multiple neurotransmitters are involved in the neural connections to and from the hypothalamus. These include noradrenergic projections from the medulla, pons and locus ceruleus, serotenergic projections from the midbrain raphe and dopaminergic neurons from the limbic system. The retinal connection to the hypothalamus mediates visual influences on neuroendocrine rhythms through melatonin. Endogenous opioids also influence hypothalamic function.

Several intrinsic **neural signals** relevant to reproduction are generated within the hypothalamus itself. These arise from what has been called the **pulse generator** for gonadotropin-releasing hormone (GnRH) and from dopaminergic neurons that project into the median eminence of the hypothalamus. Electrical recordings from the mediobasal hypothalamus reveal a synchronous increase in neuronal activity that corresponds to each pulse of LH released from the anterior pituitary. At baseline, GnRH is secreted from the hypothalamus in pulses with a frequency of one pulse per hour. This frequency changes throughout the human menstrual cycle. Dopaminergic signals travel via dopaminergic neurons from the hypothalamus to the pituitary stalk. Similar pathways also project from the hypothalamus back to the limbic system.

The **neuroendocrine signals** generated within the hypothalamus are mediated by peptide-releasing factors that travel through the hypothalamic–pituitary portal system to their site of action in the pituitary gland. **GnRH** is the key tropic hormone for regulating gonadotrope cell function and hence, reproduction (Chapter 2). **Thyrotropin-releasing hormone (TRH)** and **prolactin inhibitory factor (PIF)** also play roles in reproductive regulation. Those hypothalamic neuroendocrine peptides that control GH and ACTH secretion are less-directly related to reproduction.

Prolactin is unique among the pituitary hormones in that it is under tonic inhibitory control by the hypothalamus. Transection of the pituitary stalk therefore results in an increase in the production of prolactin, but a decrease in all other pituitary hormones. Prolactin inhibitory factor is none other than the neurotransmitter dopamine, which is secreted by the hypothalamic tuberoinfundibular neurons. Prolactin is also unique among the pituitary hormones in that its secretion is not regulated by classic feedback loops involving its target organs. Instead, prolactin secretion is controlled by local autocrine and paracrine factors, neurotransmitters and peripherally produced steroid hormones. The two major positive stimuli for prolactin secretion are TRH and oestradiol. TRH acts within the pituitary while oestrogen is active in both the hypothalamus and pituitary. Other stimuli for prolactin secretion include serotonin, opioids, oxytocin, histamine, neurotensin and substance P, all at the level of the hypothalamus. GnRH, vasoactive intestinal peptide (VIP) and angiotensin II promote prolactin secretion at the level of the posterior pituitary. The main reproductive function of prolactin is initiation and maintenance of lactation (Chapter 20). Prolactin

and growth hormone share significant structural similarities and both play important roles in immune function.

Thyroid disorders are very common during the reproductive years, especially in women. While few of these originate within the hypothalamus or pituitary, under- and overactivity of the thyroid gland can interfere with reproductive function. Abnormal amounts of circulating thyroid hormone can affect reproductive function via two mechanisms: direct effects of thyroid hormones on peripheral cells whose genes contain thyroid response elements or indirectly through the action of TRH on prolactin secretion. Most thyroid disease occurs because of inappropriate autoimmune recognition of the thyroid gland, resulting in either stimulation or destruction of the gland. This typically leaves the hypothalamic–pituitary axis intact. TSH secretion, like that of the gonadotropins, is under hypothalamic regulation by its releasing hormone, TRH. Products of the peripheral target organ, such as thyroxine, regulate the secretion of TRH and TSH via negative feedback on the hypothalamus and pituitary, respectively. Women with underactive thyroid glands have elevated levels of TRH and TSH and women with overactive thyroid glands have virtually undetectable TRH and TSH. As mentioned above, TRH is a very potent stimulant for prolactin release by the pituitary and therefore hypothyroidism often causes hyperprolactinaemia. Elevated levels of circulating prolactin are associated with menstrual irregularities (Chapter 32).

The posterior pituitary hormones, oxytocin and vasopressin-ADH, are cyclic nona-peptides secreted by the neurons of the supraoptic and paraventricular nuclei. Their identification and synthesis in the early 1950s represented the first concrete evidence that the hypothalamus exhibited endocrine function. Oxytocin has effects on uterine smooth muscle and special myoepithelial cells in the breast, promoting muscular contractions in the former and milk-letdown in the latter. Oxytocin may also act on the smooth muscle in the ejaculatory tract in men. Vasopressin-ADH has its greatest effects on vascular smooth muscle and on the collecting ducts of the kidney where it regulates intravascular volume and osmolality. Vasopressin-ADH may also play a role in sexual arousal.

Circadian rhythms

In humans exposed to normal day/night cycles, vital functions of the body change with a 24-h periodicity. This rhythm is known as the circadian rhythm and is entrained by environmental cues. The most important mediator of these cues is **melatonin**, a hormone secreted by the pineal gland. Melatonin is synthesized from serotonin by two enzymes known as N-acetyltransferase (NAT) and hydroxyindole-O-methyltransferase (HIOMT). Darkness activates melatonin secretion and light inhibits it. Light signals are transmitted to the pineal gland via neural pathways. These pathways pass through a **circadian oscillator in the hypothalamus**, down the spinal cord and through the superior cervical ganglion to the pineal gland. The dark-induced release of norepinephrine onto the pinealocytes activates β-adrenergic receptors that are coupled to cyclic adenosine monophosphate (cAMP) and NAT activity. Activation of this β-adrenergic sympathetic synapse stimulates melatonin secretion. Nocturnal melatonin secretion is associated with sleepiness, decreased core temperature and heart rate, and increased prolactin release. Melatonin has been implicated in the regulation of seasonal variations in fertility in regions with stark contrasts in day length, such as the Arctic and Scandinavia, where summer days and winter nights can be 20 h long. Melatonin concentrations are highest and conception rates are lowest during the months with the longest nights. The site of action for melatonin appears to be the suprachiasmatic nucleus of the hypothalamic. Here, it inhibits metabolic activity.

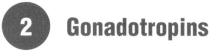

Gonadotropins

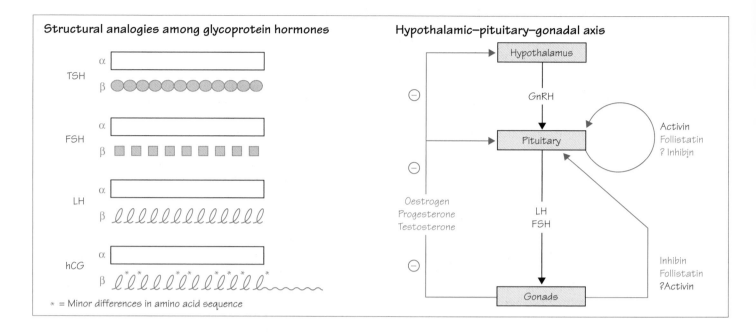

Structural analogies among glycoprotein hormones	Hypothalamic–pituitary–gonadal axis

* = Minor differences in amino acid sequence

Structure of LH and FSH

The pituitary gland produces two gonadotropins, **luteinizing hormone (LH)** and **follicle-stimulating hormone (FSH)**. Both are critical for gonadal function and reproduction in humans. Together with thyroid-stimulating hormone (TSH), LH and FSH form a major group of anterior pituitary hormones known as the glycoprotein hormones. Growth hormone and prolactin form a second group of structurally related hormones, and corticotropin, lipotropin, melanotropin and the endorphins, comprise the third group.

LH, FSH and TSH are structurally similar. They are formed by two distinct, non-covalently bound protein subunits called α and β. The pregnancy-specific gonadotropin, human chorionic gonadotropin (hCG), is a fourth glycoprotein formed of α and β chains. The α subunit for all four hormones is identical. The β subunit of each hormone differs, conferring specificity on each αβ dimer. The β chains for LH and hCG are the most similar with 82% homology. Carbohydrate side chains on both the α and β chains of LH, hCG and FSH add to structural specificity. The carbohydrate chains also influence metabolic clearance rates for the glycoprotein hormones. This effect is most dramatic with the hCG molecule. The β chain of hCG has a 24 amino acid extension at its C-terminus that contains four O-linked polysaccharides. This sugar-laden 'tail' dramatically slows the clearance of hCG. By prolonging its half-life, the effects of small amounts of this glycoprotein are dramatically enhanced. This characteristic is very important in early pregnancy recognition and maintenance (Chapters 17 and 18).

Regulation of FSH and LH

The biosynthesis and secretion of FSH and LH are tightly controlled within the reproductive cycle. Gonadotrope function is modulated by a hypothalamic factor (**gonadotropin-releasing hormone, GnRH**), pituitary factors (autocrine regulation) and gonadal feedback (reproductive steroids and peptides). There are multiple ways in which FSH

and LH can be regulated, including alterations in gene transcription, mRNA stabilization, rate of protein subunit synthesis, post-translational glycosylation and changes in the number of gonadotropin-secreting cells.

The hypothalamic decapeptide, **GnRH**, is synthesized within the arcuate nucleus of the medial basal hypothalamus and the preoptic area of the anterior hypothalamus. GnRH is transported down the axons of these specialized neuroendocrine cells through the median eminence of the hypothalamus where it is released into the portal blood system that bathes the anterior pituitary (Chapter 1). Unlike most hormones, GnRH is normally released in a pulsatile fashion. The 'pulse generator' appears to reside within the median basal hypothalamus and may be localized to the GnRH-secreting neurons themselves. The mechanism by which pulsatile GnRH release controls gonadotropin synthesis and secretion remains poorly defined. It is known that GnRH pulse frequency is most rapid in the follicular phase, slightly slower in the early luteal phase and slowest in the late luteal phase of the female menstrual cycle. In general, rapid pulse frequencies favour LH secretion and slower pulse frequencies favour FSH release. Slow pulses in the late luteal phase allow FSH increases that are essential for initiation of the subsequent menstrual cycle. The relationship between pulse frequency and LH and FSH secretion appears to exist in both women and men. Continuous GnRH release inhibits gonadotrope function.

Inhibin and **activin** are closely related peptides produced by the ovary, testes, pituitary gland and placenta that influence gonadotrope function. As suggested by their names, inhibin decreases gonadotrope function and activin stimulates it. Inhibin and activin are closely related peptides formed from common α and β subunits. Inhibin is formed of one α subunit linked to either of two highly homologous β subunits to form inhibin A ($\alpha\beta_A$) or inhibin B ($\alpha\beta_B$). Activin is composed of three combinations of the β subunits: activin A ($\beta_A\beta_A$), activin AB ($\beta_A\beta_B$) and activin B ($\beta_B\beta_B$). Activin is a member of the transforming growth factor β (TGF-β) superfamily of growth and differentiation factors that include TGF-β, Müllerian-inhibiting substance (MIS) and bone morphogenic proteins. **Follistatin** is structurally unrelated to either inhibin or activin. It is a highly glycosylated pituitary peptide that inhibits gonadotrope function but at one-third the potency of inhibin. All three of these peptides have their major influence on the expression of the FSH-β gene. Of these peptides, inhibin appears to be the most biologically important regulator of the FSH gene, directly suppressing its activity. The other two peptides appear to act within the pituitary cells through locally released second messengers or autocrine peptides. Activin B stimulates FSH release. Activins also affect the gonads directly by increasing the activity of the aromatase enzyme in the ovary and stimulating proliferation of spermatogonia in the testes.

Gonadal steroids exert negative feedback control over FSH and LH synthesis and secretion. Oestrogen, androgen and progesterone receptors are present in the gonadotropin-secreting cells of the pituitary and in some neurons in the hypothalamus. In the pituitary, the gonadal steroids appear to affect the transcription rate of the genes coding for FSH-β, LH-β and the common α subunit. While there is some evidence that steroids can act at the level of the hypothalamic pulse generator, gonadal steroid hormone receptors do not appear to be present in the GnRH-containing cells of the arcuate nucleus.

There is one important exception to the generally inhibitory effect of gonadal steroids on gonadotrope function. In certain situations, oestrogen exerts positive feedback on gonadotropin secretion. This is critical to produce the midcycle LH surge in women (Chapter 15) and requires a sustained (>48 h) elevation in circulating oestradiol. Oestrogen-induced stimulation involves both gonadotropin gene expression in the pituitary and GnRH pulse frequency in the hypothalamus.

Mechanism of action of gonadotropins

The **receptors** for the glycoprotein hormones are located in the plasma membranes of their target cells in the gonads. There are distinct FSH and LH receptors. The latter also bind the closely related hCG molecule. Although these receptors are normally present in very low concentrations on the cell surface, they have high specificity and affinity for their ligands. The interactions between the glycoprotein dimer and the receptor lead to conformational change in the receptor. This then activates a membrane-associated **G protein-coupled signalling system**. Other important members of the G protein-coupled receptor family include receptors for GnRH and for α-adrenergic, β-adrenergic and dopaminergic compounds. Within this receptor superfamily, receptor binding is an event distinct from receptor activation and downstream intracellular signalling. These processes may be differentially affected by disease states.

G proteins are a subset of regulatory guanosine triphosphate (GTP)-binding proteins that activate adenylate cyclase and increase intracellular cAMP production. The conformational change induced by binding of the gonadotropin to a G protein-coupled receptor on the cell surface results in the replacement of an intracellular subunit of the G protein with GTP. The dissociated G protein subunit ($G_{s\alpha}$) then activates adenylate cyclase to produce cAMP. Increased cAMP activates the intracellular protein kinase A pathway that, in turn, modulates the function of a number of cell processes by protein phosphorylation. In the ovary and testes, this increase in cAMP is responsible for gonadal steroidogenesis and gametogenesis (Chapter 3).

Although the cAMP pathway is the principal mediator of both FSH and LH receptor activity, activation of the protein kinase C system can also occur. This involves activation of a different G protein subunit, G_q, by LH/hCG binding to the LH receptor. G_q then activates phospholipase C, which digests membrane lipids, producing two intracellular messengers: 1,2-diacylglycerol (DAG) and inositol triphosphate ($InsP_3$). DAG activates protein kinase C while $InsP_3$ releases calcium from the endoplasmic reticulum into the intracellular space.

In addition to activating specific intracellular signalling processes, binding of the gonadotropin to its receptor also initiates a regulatory function called **desensitization**. Desensitization reduces the cell's responsiveness to ongoing stimulation. In the first phase of desensitization, the gonadotropin receptor becomes 'uncoupled' from its downstream activity so that it no longer activates adenylate cyclase. In the second, slower phase of desensitization, the degradation rate for the receptors is increased. This latter process is called 'down-regulation'.

Both LH and FSH receptors are present in the plasma membranes of granulosa cells in the ovary and Sertoli cells in the testes. Ovarian thecal cells and testicular Leydig cells only display LH receptors. In addition to regulating steroidogenesis and gametogenesis, gonadotropins regulate expression of their own receptors in a dose-dependent fashion. FSH also induces LH/hCG receptor formation in granulosa and Sertoli cells.

A carefully defined sequence of hormonal changes is necessary for normal follicular development and ovulation in the ovary (Chapter 13). Initiation of follicular growth occurs independent of gonadotropin stimulation; however, unless gonadotropins are present, these follicles will rapidly undergo atresia. Because theca cells lack FSH receptors, they only respond to LH. LH increases the production of androgen precursors in theca cells (Chapter 3). FSH causes granulosa cell proliferation around the developing follicles and oestrogen biosynthesis by these cells. FSH induces the enzyme aromatase within the granulosa cells. Aromatase converts the androgens produced in the theca cells to oestrogens in the granulosa cells. FSH also increases inhibin production by the granulosa cells prior to ovulation.

Once ovulation has occurred, the theca cells surrounding the ruptured ovarian follicle are converted to a corpus luteum. The corpus luteum responds to LH stimulation by producing progesterone. LH increases the cellular uptake of low-density lipoprotein (LDL) cholesterol by corpus luteum cells through induction of LDL receptors. It simultaneously promotes LDL conversion to progesterone by inducing the two rate-limiting enzyme complexes necessary for progesterone synthesis: P450cc and 3β-hydroxysteroid dehydrogenase, Maintenance of steroid production by the corpus luteum is LH dependent; however, the finite 14-day life span of the corpus luteum does not appear to be related to a decrease in LH stimulation. The factor(s) responsible for the demise of the corpus luteum are unknown. As the function of the corpus luteum wanes near the end of the cycle, synthesis of inhibin, oestrogen and progesterone decreases and production of FSH by the pituitary increases. This next wave of FSH production 'rescues' developing follicles from atresia.

In the male, FSH stimulates spermatogenesis within the seminiferous epithelium and production of androgen-binding protein, aromatase and inhibin by the Sertoli cells. The latter exerts negative feedback on FSH secretion by the pituitary. LH stimulates testosterone production by the Leydig cells. Testosterone promotes masculinization at peripheral target sites after local conversion to its more potent metabolite, dyhydrotestosterone (DHT).

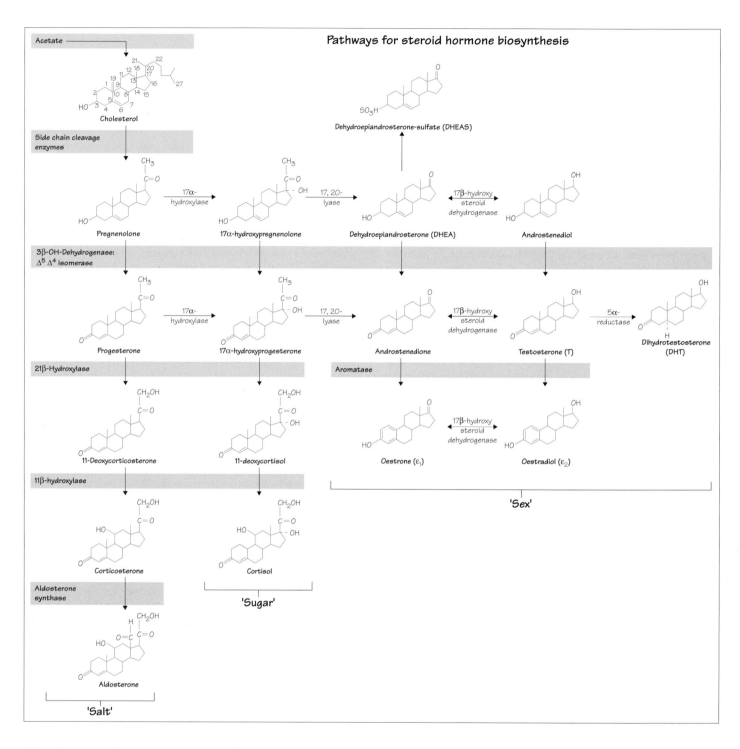

Pathways for steroid hormone biosynthesis

Cholesterol and the steroid production pathway

Cholesterol is the building block of steroid hormones. All steroid-producing organs with the exception of the placenta can synthesize cholesterol from acetate. Under most circumstances, however, local synthesis cannot meet demand and circulating cholesterol must be used. The major carriers of cholesterol in the bloodstream are the **low-density lipoproteins (LDLs)**. LDL is removed from the blood by steroidogenic cells using cell surface receptors that recognize specific surface proteins on LDL called apoproteins. Once in the cell, cholesterol is carried through a sequence of enzymatic changes to produce a final product that belongs to one of the major classes of steroid hormones: progestins, androgens, oestrogens (sex), glucocorticoids (sugar) and mineralocorticoids (salt). All steroid-producing tissues use a common sequence of

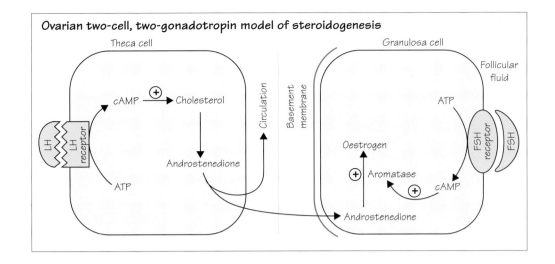

Ovarian two-cell, two-gonadotropin model of steroidogenesis

precursor molecules and enzymes. Tissue specificity is conferred by the presence or absence of specific enzymes in the sequence. For instance, the gonads differ from the adrenal glands in that ovaries and testes do not express the 21-hydroxylase or 11β-hydroxylase enzymes that are necessary to produce corticosteroids. Therefore, the gonads only produce three classes of steroids: progestins, androgens and oestrogens.

During conversion of cholesterol to steroid metabolites, the number of total carbon atoms decreases sequentially. Progestins have 21 carbons (C-21); androgens, 19 carbons (C-19); and oestrogens, 18 carbons (C-18). Thus progestins are obligatory precursors of both androgens and oestrogens. Likewise, androgens are obligatory precursors of oestrogens.

Most of the steroidogenic enzymes are members of the **cytochrome P450 class of oxidases**. A single mitochondrial protein P450scc, the cholesterol side chain cleavage enzyme, mediates all steps in the conversion of cholesterol to pregnenolone. The activity of this protein represents the rate-limiting step for the entire steroid pathway. Not surprisingly, it is also the major site of tropic hormone stimulation. Genetic mutations of P450scc are very rare and usually lethal. No steroid hormones can be produced by an individual with an inactive P450scc enzyme.

Once pregnenolone is formed, steroid production can proceed down one of two paths, through either progesterone or 17α-hydroxypregnenolone. All but two of the enzymes responsible for producing the steroid hormones are packaged within the endoplasmic reticulum, together with other members of the P450 system. The biosynthetic units are very tightly linked together, thereby ensuring that very few of the steroid intermediates leave the cell. This packaging is also highly efficient in that it can convert an entire class of steroids to another. Thus, 17,20-desmolase will convert all progestins to androgens, and aromatase will convert all androgens but dihydrotestosterone (DHT) to oestrogens.

Sites of production
Ovary
In the ovary, steroid production occurs in a **two-cell system**. Theca cells produce androgens. These diffuse into the granulosa cells where they are converted to oestrogens. Tropic hormones regulate specific steps in the sex steroid cascade. Theca cells respond to **luteinizing hormone (LH)** by increasing the number of LDL receptors and hence cholesterol entry into the cells. LH also stimulates P450scc activity, allowing increased androgen production. When these androgens diffuse into

granulosa cells, they are metabolized by aromatase into oestrogens. **Follicle-stimulating hormone (FSH)** induces the activity of aromatase in the granulosa cell, thereby increasing the conversion of androgens to oestrogens. The single aromatase gene has many promoter sites. These are responsive to cytokines, cyclic nucleotides, gonadotropins, glucocorticoids and growth factors.

Testes
In the testes, androgen production occurs largely in the Leydig cells under the influence of LH. Androgens produced in the Leydig cells either enter the bloodstream directly or diffuse into nearby Sertoli cells. Sertoli cells can convert androgens to oestrogens using aromatase or reduce them to dihydrotestosterone via 5α-reductase. Because the specific cell types within the differentiated male and female gonads have common embryonic origins (Chapter 6), the mechanisms for steroid production in the testes very much parallel those in the ovary.

Adrenals
Sex hormone production by the adrenals occurs largely as a by-product of corticosteroid biosynthesis. The contribution of adrenal sex steroids to the total pool of circulating sex steroids is typically small, although there are several important exceptions. The ovaries of postmenopausal women no longer produce significant amounts of steroid hormones so adrenal androgen production can become clinically significant. In pregnancy, the placenta cannot synthesize cholesterol from acetate. Rather, it relies on adrenal androgens of both maternal and fetal origin to make oestrogens.

With the exception of P450scc, inherited defects in any of the enzymes involved in steroidogenesis are associated with clinical syndromes resulting either from accumulation of a precursor product or absence of a key end-product. For example, an inherited deficiency of the enzyme 21-hydroxylase in the adrenal gland will lead to a deficiency in adrenal cortisol production. Low cortisol levels feed back to promote enhanced production of adrenal glucocorticoids. The enzymatic block, however, results in an accumulation of precursor progestins, some of which will be shunted down functional androgen biosynthetic pathways. If the 21-hydroxylase deficiency occurs in a female fetus, the increase in androgen production may cause masculinization of the external genitalia, known as congenital adrenal hyperplasia syndrome (Chapter 27). Similarly, disorders of male sexual differentiation and development may result from genetic defects in androgen production (Chapter 26).

4 Steroid hormone mechanism of action and metabolism

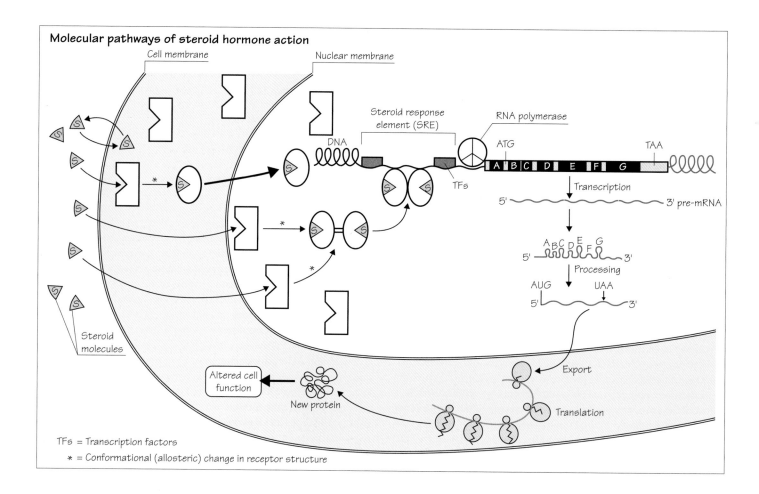

Molecular pathways of steroid hormone action

TFs = Transcription factors

∗ = Conformational (allosteric) change in receptor structure

Mechanisms of steroid action

Steroid hormones exert their effects via a unifying basic mechanism: the induction of new protein synthesis in their target cells. These induced proteins may be hormones themselves or other molecules important to cell function, such as enzymes. It is the newly synthesized proteins that are ultimately responsible for steroid hormone activity.

Once a steroid hormone is secreted by its endocrine gland of origin, 95–98% of it circulates in the bloodstream bound to a specific transport protein. The remaining 2–5% is free to diffuse into all cells. Once inside the cell, a steroid can only produce responses in cells that have **specific intracellular receptors** for that hormone. Specific receptor binding is key to the action of steroids in their target tissues. Thus, oestrogen receptors are found in the brain and in target cells specific to female reproduction, such as the uterus and breast. Facial hair follicles and penile erectile tissue contain androgen receptors. Glucocorticoid receptors are found in all cells because glucocorticoids are necessary to regulate global functions like metabolism and stress.

All members of the major classes of sex steroids (e.g. androgens, oestrogens and progestins) act through a similar sequence of events to exert cellular responses. These include: (i) transfer of the steroid into the nucleus; (ii) intranuclear receptor binding; (iii) alterations in receptor conformation that convert the receptor from an inactive to an active form; (iv) binding of the steroid-receptor complex to regulatory elements on deoxyribonucleic acid (DNA); (v) transcription and synthesis of new messenger ribonucleic acid (mRNA); and (vi) translation of mRNA with new protein synthesis in the cell. The mechanisms of action of glucocorticoids and mineralocorticoids differ from those of the sex steroids. Glucocorticoids and mineralocorticoids bind to their receptors in the cell cytoplasm. Hormone-receptor complexes are subsequently transported to the nucleus where they bind to the DNA.

There are three important structural domains in each steroid hormone receptor that correspond to the molecule's three functions: (i) steroid hormone binding; (ii) DNA binding; and (iii) promotion of gene transcription. It is therefore not surprising that all steroid hormone receptors have remarkable structural similarities at the copy DNA (cDNA) level. The receptors for thyroid hormone, vitamin D and vitamin A also have similar DNA binding domains. Together with the sex hormone receptors, these receptors form a 'superfamily' of nuclear receptors in which the thyroid hormone and vitamin A and D receptors are thought to be the most evolutionarily primitive. The latter three receptors are highly conserved, likely a result of their importance in early embryonic development. Glucocorticoid and progesterone receptors arose more recently in evolution. Their actions are less global, regulating acute metabolic changes in highly differentiated cells.

Expression of genes regulated by steroid hormones is controlled by four specific elements called (i) promoters, (ii) steroid-responsive enhancers, (iii) silencers and (iv) hormone-independent enhancers. Steroid-responsive enhancers are DNA binding sites for activated steroid-receptor complexes and are known as steroid response elements (SREs). SREs are a very important component of hormone-responsive genes: they determine steroid specificity.

Agonists and antagonists

Steroid hormone potency depends on a combination of the affinity of the receptor for the hormone or drug, the affinity of the hormone–receptor complex for the SRE, and the efficiency of the activated hormone–receptor complex in regulating gene transcription. Molecules with high affinities for a receptor and whose subsequent hormone–receptor complex has high affinity for an SRE lead to prolonged occupancy of the SRE and sustained gene transcription. Such molecules act as agonists for the parent compound. Other molecules may have a high affinity for a receptor, but the hormone–receptor complex binds inefficiently to the SRE. Still others occupy the steroid receptor in a way that allows them to bind to the SRE but prevents RNA polymerase from coupling with factors necessary for gene transcription. The latter act as antagonists to the parent compound. An example of a compound with mixed agonist/antagonist properties is the drug tamoxifen. **Tamoxifen** is an antioestrogen that acts as a potent antagonist to the oestrogen receptor in breast tissue and as an agonist in uterus and bone. Such tissue-specific effects are dependent upon specific silencers and hormone-independent enhancers present in each tissue. Another widely used agonist/antagonist is the non-steroidal compound clomiphene citrate. **Clomiphene** can be used to induce ovulation, although its actions are complex. Clomiphene's interactions with oestrogen receptors in the pituitary gland and hypothalamus result in binding of receptors, but without subsequent efficient stimulation of oestrogen-associated gene transcription. The hypothalamus senses this as a hypo-oestrogenic state and GnRH pulse frequency increases. Pituitary follicle-stimulating hormone (FSH) production is stimulated and increased FSH release drives ovarian production of oestrogen. Oestrogen acts locally to recruit ovarian follicles for ovulation. When clomiphene is stopped, the hypothalamic oestrogen receptors are again available for oestrogen binding and appropriate SRE responses. The hypothalamus is able to respond normally to the high concentrations of circulating oestrogen from the ovaries and an ovulatory luteinizing hormone (LH) surge occurs (Chapter 15).

Steroids in the circulation

Steroid hormones are transported in the bloodstream bound to specific proteins. Protein-bound hormone does not traverse the plasma membrane of the cell. Nearly 70% of circulating testosterone and oestradiol is bound to a β globulin known as **sex hormone-binding globulin (SHBG)**. Another 30% is loosely bound to albumin, leaving only 1–2% unbound and capable of entering cells. SHBG binds all other oestrogens and androgens to varying degrees; less than 10% of any steroid is free in the bloodstream. Pregnancy, oestrogen and hyperthyroidism all increase SHBG synthesis. Androgens, progestins, corticoids and growth hormone all decrease SHBG. Weight gain can also decrease SHBG through an insulin-mediated effect on its synthesis. In keeping with the law of mass action, changes in the concentration of SHBG will affect the amount of free, unbound circulating steroid. Changes in SHBG will therefore affect the biological action of steroids by altering the amount available to cells.

Unlike the other sex steroids, progesterone is carried in the blood by a glycoprotein, corticosteroid-binding globulin (CBG). CBG is also known as transcortin. As suggested by its name, it binds and carries glucocorticoids.

Steroid metabolism

With the exception of the progestins, androgens are obligatory precursors of all other steroid hormones. Therefore, androgens are made in all steroid-producing tissues including the testis, ovary and adrenal gland. The major circulating androgen in men is testosterone that is produced by the testes. **Testosterone is the most potent androgen**. Its hormonal action is produced either directly through binding to the androgen receptor or indirectly after **conversion to dihydrotestosterone (DHT)** within the target tissue. Testosterone acts directly on the internal genital tract in male fetuses during sexual differentiation (Chapter 7) and on skeletal muscle to promote growth. DHT acts on the genital tracts of male fetuses to stimulate differentiation of the external genitalia. In adult men, DHT acts locally to maintain masculinized external genitalia and secondary sexual characteristics such as facial and pubic hair. Other major circulating androgens in men include androstenedione, androstenediol, dehydroepiandrosterone (DHEA) and dehydroepiandrosterone sulfate (DHEA-S).

All of the above androgens, including testosterone and DHT, can be found in the circulation of women. With the exception of androstenedione, the concentrations of the androgens are considerably less in women than in men. Androstenedione is unique in that only about 4% of it is bound to SHBG in the circulation in women. The remainder is bound more loosely to albumin. Circulating androstenedione functions largely as a prohormone and is converted within target tissues to testosterone, oestrone and oestradiol.

Oestradiol (E_2) is the major oestrogen secreted by the ovary. Oestrone (E_1) is also secreted by the ovary in significant amounts. Oestriol (E_3), by contrast, is not produced in the ovary at all. Oestriol is produced from oestradiol and oestrone in peripheral tissues and from androgen in the placenta; it is considered a less active 'metabolite' of the more potent oestrogens. Direct conversion of androgens into oestrone can occur in skin and adipose tissue. This has important clinical implications in the obese female. In all women, the daily production of the prohormone androstenedione is 10 times higher than estradiol. In obese women, conversion of androgens to oestrone in adipose tissue can become a major source of excessive amounts of circulating oestrogen.

The adrenal gland is an important source of sex steroids in both men and women. Androstenedione, DHEA and DHEA-S are the major circulating androgens of adrenal origin and adrenal androgen production follows a circadian rhythm that parallels cortisol secretion. Adrenal androgens assume an important role in the postmenopausal woman. In the absence of ovarian oestrogen production, adrenal androgens act as a major source for oestrogen precursors.

The most abundant progestin in the circulation is **progesterone**. The ovary, testis, placenta and adrenal gland can all produce progesterone. 17-Hydroxyprogesterone of adrenal and ovarian origin represents the other major circulating progestin. Both progestins are largely bound by transcortin.

Steroid excretion

Steroids are excreted in urine and bile. Prior to elimination, most active steroids are conjugated as either sulfates or glucuronides. Some sulfated conjugates such as DHEA-S are actively secreted. These conjugated hormones can serve as precursors to active hormone metabolites in target tissues that have the enzymes to hydrolyze the ester bonds involved in the conjugation.

5 Reproductive genetics

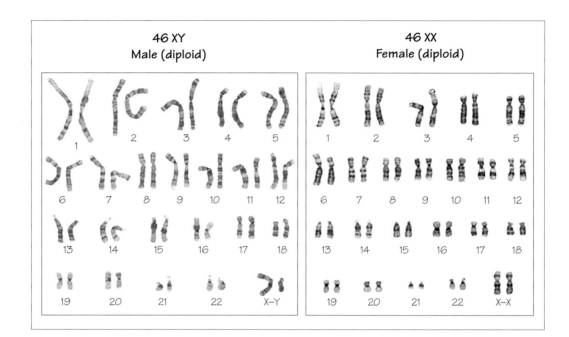

Chromosomes

Human chromosomes are complex structures consisting of deoxyribonucleic acid (DNA), ribonucleic acid (RNA) and protein. Each single helix of DNA is bounded at each end with a telomere, and has a centromere somewhere along the length of the chromosome. The telomere protects the ends of the chromosome during DNA replication. Telomere shortening is associated with aging. The centromere is the site at which the mitotic spindle will attach and is necessary for proper segregation of the chromosomes during cell division. The centromere divides the chromosome into two arms, identified as p (petit) for the short arm and q for the long arm. The centromere can be positioned anywhere along the arm of the chromosome and its location has been used to group like chromosomes together as central (metacentric), distal (acrocentric) or others (submetacentric). The length of the chromosome plus the position of its centromere are used to identify individual chromosomes within the 22 pairs of autosomes and one pair of sex chromosomes. The chromosomes are numbered in descending order of size; 1 is the largest. The single exception to this rule is chromosomes 21 and 22: 22 is larger than 21. Because of the historical convention of associating Down syndrome with trisomy 21, this chromosome pair was not renamed when the size difference became apparent.

A **karyotype** is a display of chromosomes ordered from 1 to 22 plus the sex chromosomes, with each chromosome oriented so that the p arm is on top. Females have a 46XX karyotype and males a 46XY karyotype.

Mitosis and meiosis

These are two distinct types of cell divisions, with several common features. The first is the need to duplicate the entire chromosome content of the cell prior to division. Both also use the cell machinery of the parent cell to make the DNA, RNA and new proteins that will participate in the cell division. Finally, both processes rely on using the mitotic spindle to separate the chromosomes into the two poles of the cell that are destined to become the progeny of that cell. Mitosis and meiosis differ in that duplicated chromosomes behave differently after DNA replication. In mitosis, there is no difference on total chromosome content between parent and daughter cells; in meiosis, the chromosome number of the daughter cells is eventually reduced from 46 to 23, which is necessary to convert the diploid germ cell precursors originating in the embryo into haploid ($1n$) germ cells. These haploid germ cells will produce a new diploid organism at fertilization. Meiosis promotes exchange of genetic material through chromatid crossing over; mitosis does not.

During the **interphase** preceding cell division, the DNA for each chromosome is duplicated to $4n$. Thus, each chromosome consists of two identical **chromatids** joined at the centromere.

In mitosis, the chromosomes first shorten and thicken and the nucleoli and nuclear membrane break down (**prophase**). During **metaphase**, a mitotic spindle forms between the two centrioles of the cell and all chromosomes line up on its equator. The centromere for each chromosome splits and one chromatid from each chromosome migrates to the polar ends of the mitotic spindle (**anaphase**). Finally, in **telophase**, new nucleoli and nuclear membranes form, the parent cell divides into two daughter cells and the mitotic spindle is disassembled. Two genetically identical cells now exist in place of the parent cell. **Mitosis is considered a non-sexual or vegetative form of reproduction**.

Meiosis involves two sequential cell divisions, again beginning with the 4N DNA produced in interphase. In prophase of the first division (**prophase 1**), several specific and recognizable events occur. In the **leptotene** stage, the chromosomes become barely visible as long thin structures. Homologous pairs of chromosomes then come to lie side by side along parts of their length, forming tetrads (**zygotene** stage). The chromosomes thicken and shorten, much as they do in mitotic prophase (**pachytene** stage); however, the pairing that occurred in the zygotene stage permits **synapsis**, **crossing-over** and **chromatid exchange** to take place. In the **diplotene/diakinesis** stage, the chromosomes shorten even more.

Mitosis and meiosis in human cells

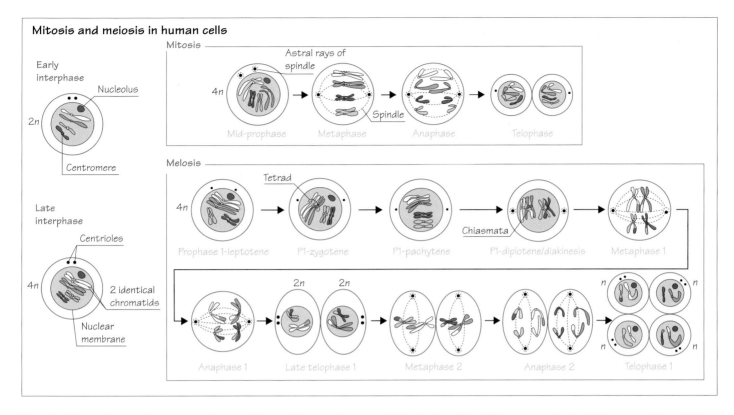

The paired homologous chromosomes show evidence of the crossing-over and chromatid exchange, displaying characteristic chiasmata that join the chromosome arms. Loops and unusual shapes within the chromosomes may be apparent at this stage. In **metaphase 1** of meiosis, the nuclear membrane breaks down and the joined pairs of homologous chromosomes line up at the equator of the spindle apparatus. One of each pair of homologous chromosomes then moves to each end of the cell along the spindle (**anaphase 1**). Nuclear membranes may form, yielding two haploid daughter cells with 23 $2n$ chromosomes in **telophase 1**. In the second meiotic division, these haploid cells divide as if in mitosis. This second division produces four haploid cells each containing 23 $1n$ chromosomes. **Unlike the cells produced in mitosis, these daughter germ cells are genetically unique and different from the parent cells because of the genetic exchanges that took place in the diplotene stage.** Haploid germ cells will participate in sexual reproduction in which a sperm cell and oocyte come together to form a new diploid zygote.

While the sequence of events in meiosis during spermatogenesis and oogenesis is basically the same, there are several important differences. In the prepubertal male, primordial germ cells are arrested in interphase. At puberty, these cells are reactivated to enter rounds of mitoses in the basal compartment of the seminiferous tubule. These reactivated cells are known as spermatogonial stem cells. From this reservoir of stem cells, spermatogonia emerge and divide several times again to produce a 'clone' of spermatogonia with identical genotypes. All the spermatogonia from the clone then enter meiosis 1 and 2 to produce unique haploid sperm. New stem cells are constantly entering the spermatogenic cycle (Chapter 9) and thus the sperm supply is constantly renewing itself. Because of the relatively short time for spermatocytes to progress through meiosis and because of the tremendous competition among spermatozoa to reach the single oocyte within the female tract, fertilization of an egg by an aneuploid sperm is far rarer than the converse.

In contrast to the testis, the ovary of a female at birth contains all the germ cells it will ever have. These oocytes remain arrested in prophase 1 of meiosis until the LH surge at ovulation initiates metaphase 1. Thus, the duplicated genetic material within the oocyte exists paired with its homologous chromosome for 10–50 years before the cell is called upon to divide. For this reason alone, oocytes are much more prone to chromosome abnormalities than are sperm.

Non-disjunction

This is the failure of a chromosome pair to separate during meiosis, and can occur at either meiosis 1 or 2. When a single chromosome is involved, the aneuploid zygote is either **monosomic** or **trisomic** for the chromosome pair that failed to divide properly. With the exception of monosomy X or Turner syndrome, monosomic embryos are uniformly miscarried (Chapter 36). Most trisomic fetuses are also miscarried; only three (trisomy 13, 18 and 21) are reported among live births. If all the chromosomes are present in multiples other than $2n$, the embryo or fetus is **polyploid**.

Imprinting

Although it is critical that the zygote has $2n$ chromosomes, it is also important that one set of chromosomes comes from each parent. Dermoid cysts and hydatidiform moles (gestational trophoblastic disease) (Chapter 44) each have all 46 chromosomes from a single parent. Cytogenetic studies of these entities have shown the importance of imprinting in early embryonic development. Imprinting is the process by which specific genes are methylated so that they can no longer be transcribed. Normal embryonic development requires that one set of genes be maternally imprinted and a second paternally. Otherwise, important steps in development will not occur and the zygote cannot form normally. For instance, two sets of maternally imprinted genes are present in dermoid tumours of the ovary, resulting in development of disorganized fetal tissues without any supporting placenta or fetal membranes. Conversely, two sets of paternally imprinted genes are present in hydatidiform moles. In these cases, dysplastic trophoblast develops, but a fetus does not.

6 Gonadal development in the embryo

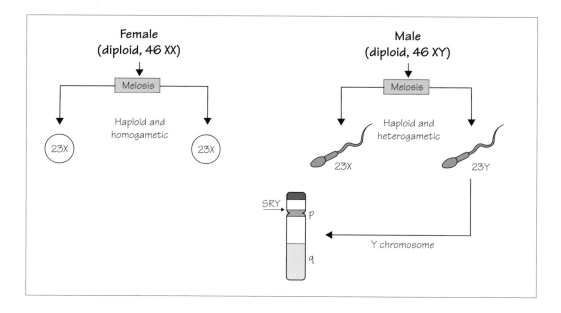

Role of sex chromatin in reproductive development

All mammalian females are homogametic and represent the 'default' pathway in sexual differentiation. Homogametic animals produce gametes with a single chromosomal constitution. In humans, all normal oocytes from genetic females will carry 22 autosomes and an X chromosome (22X). Mammalian embryos of both genetic sexes are bathed in relatively large amounts of placental oestrogen during development. In the absence of specific factors regulated by a single gene on the Y chromosome, embryos will develop into a female phenotype. The human female, like all mammalian females, represents the fundamental or undifferentiated phenotypic sex.

All mammalian males are heterogametic. They produce gametes with both 22X and 22Y chromosome complements. Males are considered the differentiated phenotypic sex. With few exceptions, any individual that carries a specific piece of the Y chromosome will develop a testis and a male phenotype. This segment of the Y chromosome has been called the **sex-determining region of the Y chromosome (SRY)**. Specific instruction from the SRY region of the Y chromosome directs the undifferentiated gonad to become a testis. **Without the presence of SRY, a fetus will develop along the default or female phenotypic pathway.**

The Y chromosome is much smaller than the X and very little of its DNA is available for RNA synthesis. Many of the genes that control testicular development from the undifferentiated gonad are therefore located on other chromosomes, including autosomes and the X chromosome. The Y chromosome does, however, contain a specific, single-copy gene that determines testicular differentiation. This gene is located on the short arm of the chromosome within SRY and appears to activate genes on these other chromosomes.

Evidence for the importance of SRY comes from both clinical and experimental research results. Examination of the DNA sequences of women with XY karyotypes has revealed that a single locus within the Y chromosome must be present and intact for an individual to have a testis. Absence of, or damage to this DNA sequence in individuals with an otherwise intact 46XY male chromosomal content results in ovarian development and a phenotypic female. Likewise, examination of the DNA sequences of phenotypic men with XX karyotypes will reveal the aberrant presence of SRY sequences.

Gonadal differentiation

Gonadal development begins in the human at the 4th embryonic (6th menstrual) week in parallel with the formation of the ventral body wall. The first step in gonadal development is the migration of undifferentiated primordial germ cells from their site of formation in the yolk sac. These germ cells arise from the endoderm lining the yolk sac; they detach themselves and migrate dorsally along the yolk stalk, midgut and dorsal mesentery to reach the genital ridges. The genital ridges lie on the medial aspect of the mesonephric ridge that will contribute to the developing kidney. Over the next 2 weeks the primordial germ cells mitose repeatedly, forming a vast population of precursor gametes. Failure of these germ cells to develop and populate the genital ridges at this time will result in complete failure of gonadal formation.

When germ cells reach the coelomic epithelium lining the genital ridge, cellular contact causes the coelomic epithelia to differentiate into a primitive germinal epithelium. The germ cells become embedded in the primitive germinal epithelium during this process of differentiation. This combination of germinal epithelia and germ cells forms the sex cords. The connection of the sex cords to the coelomic wall (gonadal surface) is maintained at this point. The gonads are now histologically distinct, bipotent organs that may become testes or ovaries. Inappropriate or incomplete developmental signals during this stage can result in the rare condition of hermaphroditism. Hermaphrodites have a discrepancy between their genetic sex and their gonadal sex.

In a genetic male, gene products directed by activation of the SRY locus on the Y chromosome now cause the undifferentiated sex cords to

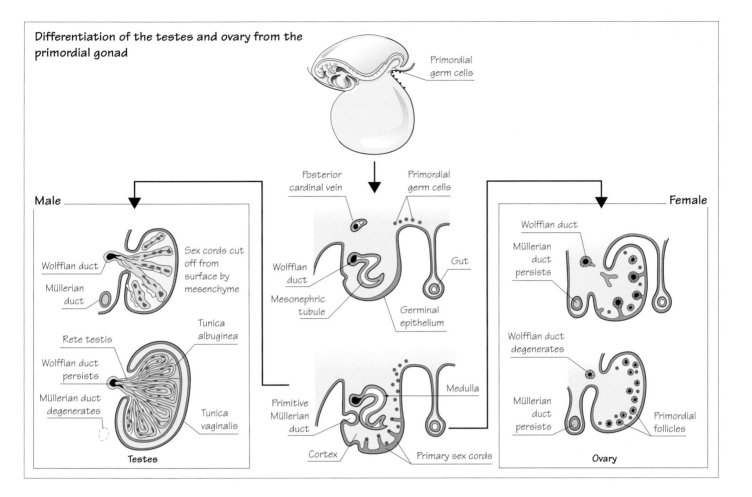

Differentiation of the testes and ovary from the primordial gonad

Male

- Wolffian duct
- Müllerian duct
- Sex cords cut off from surface by mesenchyme
- Rete testis
- Wolffian duct persists
- Müllerian duct degenerates
- Tunica albuginea
- Tunica vaginalis

Testes

- Primordial germ cells
- Posterior cardinal vein
- Primordial germ cells
- Wolffian duct
- Mesonephric tubule
- Gut
- Germinal epithelium
- Primitive Müllerian duct
- Medulla
- Cortex
- Primary sex cords

Female

- Wolffian duct
- Müllerian duct persists
- Wolffian duct degenerates
- Müllerian duct persists
- Primordial follicles

Ovary

---

enlarge, split and begin to form the **primitive testis**. Subepithelial mesenchyme arises between the germinal epithelium and the sex cords and cuts the cords off from the gonadal surface. The sex cords are now housed within the inner portion of the gonad—**the testicular medulla**. The primordial germ cells within the sex cords begin to differentiate into immature sperm cells called **spermatogonia**. The supporting sex cord cells form precursor **Sertoli cells**.

Ovarian differentiation occurs about 2 weeks later than testicular development. Initially, the sex cords of the developing ovary continue to proliferate while maintaining their connection with the gonadal surface. The germ cells begin to differentiate into primordial **oocytes** called oogonia within follicles. The epithelium surrounding the oogonia differentiates into **granulosa cells**. Subepithelial mesenchyme then invades the gonad and breaks up the sex cords, isolating the follicles. This mesenchyme will become the ovarian stroma. Unlike the testis, developing gametes are now housed in the outer portion of the gonad—**the ovarian cortex**.

The ovary and testes can be histologically distinguished from each other by the 8th embryonic (10th menstrual) week of pregnancy. The progeny of the germinal epithelium are now apparent as Sertoli cells in the male and granulosa cells in the female. Similarities between males and females in the endocrine function of these cells stem from their common ancestry. The mesenchyme arising beneath the germinal epithelium in the testis is the anlagen of testicular interstitial cells, also known as **Leydig cells**. The mesenchyme arising beneath the germinal epithelium of the ovary is the anlagen of ovarian stroma or **thecal cells**. Functional similarities in these two cell types will also be seen in the mature glands.

Once the undifferentiated gonad begins to develop into either ovary or testis, the remainder of sexual differentiation is dependent on secretory products of the testes only. In the absence of these specific testicular secretions, the phenotype that develops is completely female. The ovary and its secretory products do not contribute to the development of the uterus, Fallopian tubes or vulva.

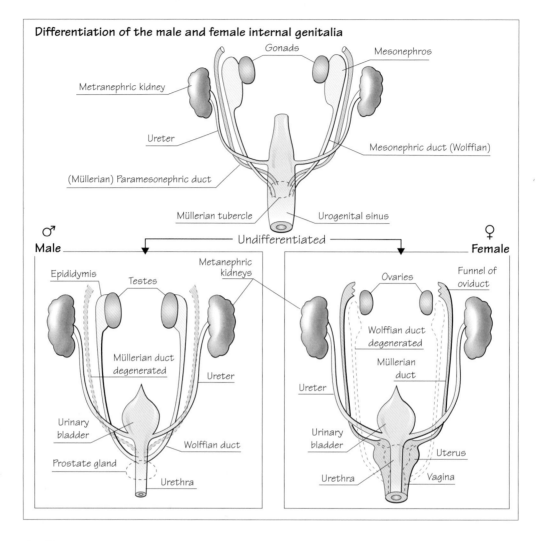

Differentiation of the male and female internal genitalia

Internal genitalia

Unlike the bipotential gonads and external genitalia, the male and female internal genitalia arise from separate duct systems. Development of these structures occurs in parallel and in close physical proximity with the developing urinary system. Both begin to occur at about 4 embryonic (6 menstrual) weeks. The primordial kidney (mesonephros) is composed of tubules and a duct known as the **mesonephric or Wolffian duct**. The Wolffian duct grows out from the tubules toward the urogenital sinus. The mesonephric tubules make contact with the primitive sex cords just as the gonad begins to differentiate. Simultaneously, an inpocketing of the coelomic epithelium near the lateral edge of the mesonephric ridge forms the paramesonephric or **Müllerian duct**. As kidney development proceeds (metanephric stage), the mesonephric structures will become totally incorporated into the reproductive tract and lose their urinary function. The Wolffian and Müllerian ducts are primordia for the internal organs of reproduction in the male and female, respectively. In each sex, the other duct system typically disappears by the 3rd fetal month, leaving behind only unimportant vestiges.

In the normal male embryo, the secretion of a peptide called Müllerian-inhibiting substance (MIS) occurs under the direction of SRY. MIS is secreted by cells that will become Sertoli cells in the adult testis. It causes the Müllerian duct to degenerate. Testosterone is produced by those testicular cells destined to become Leydig cells in the adult. Testosterone directs development of the **Wolffian duct system** to form the **epididymis**, **vas deferens** and **seminal vesicles**. In contrast to the adult, testosterone production by the embryonic testes is controlled not by the hypothalamic–pituitary system, but by the placental hormone human chorionic gonadotropin (hCG).

The absence of MIS in the female embryo permits the Müllerian system to persist. Upon reaching the urogenital sinus, the Müllerian ducts induce the formation of a vaginal plate. Contact of the Müllerian ducts with the vaginal plate also initiates the fusion of the ducts to form the body of the uterus. The Müllerian ducts will form the **Fallopian tubes**, **uterus** and **upper one-third of the vagina**. Failure of the Müllerian ducts to develop or fuse completely can cause uterine and cervical anomalies. In the absence of testosterone, the Wolffian system regresses. A vestige of the Wolffian duct, known as Gartner's duct, persists in its length from the ovary to the hymen. Clinically apparent cysts may form anywhere along Gartner's duct.

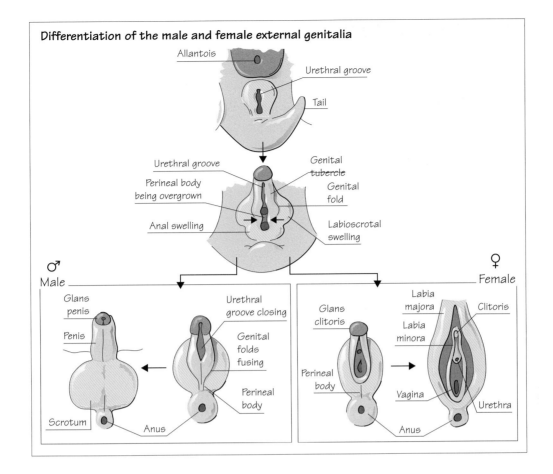

Differentiation of the male and female external genitalia

External genitalia

Like the primordial gonads, the anlagen of the external genitalia are bipotential. In the 8th embryonic (10th menstrual) week, a urogenital slit, a genital tubercle, two lateral genital folds and two labioscrotal swellings become apparent as precursors to the external genitalia.

While differentiation of the internal Wolffian duct system is testosterone dependent, the primordial external genital structures require the presence of DHT to differentiate into recognizably male structures. The source of the DHT is testicular testosterone, converted locally to DHT in the primordial external genitalia. In the presence of DHT, the lobes of the prostate gland grow out from the seminal colliculus where the urethra is developing from the bladder. The genital folds fuse to form the **penis** around the elongating urethra. The labioscrotal swellings enlarge and fuse to form the **scrotum**.

Descent of the testes from the abdomen into the scrotum is an androgen-dependent event during which the testes are pulled downward by a fibrous cord anchored to the developing scrotum—the **gubernaculum**. During development, a peritoneal fold around the Wolffian and Müllerian ducts (destined to eventually become the tunica vaginalis) connects to the genital swelling, and the gubernaculum forms

Most of the **prostate gland** develops from the same primordial area of the urogenital sinus that forms the vaginal plate in the female, making the prostate a homologue of the upper vagina. Mesenchyme in this tissue differentiates into the peripheral zone of the prostate, under the influence of **dihydrotestosterone (DHT)**. In the presence of a functional fetal testis, DHT is produced locally from testosterone by the enzyme 5α-reductase. The more central tissue in this area, which may be of Wolffian derivation, forms the central and transition zones of the prostate.

as a ridge under the peritoneum. The gubernaculum connecting the testis to the genital swelling does not grow as rapidly as the remainder of the embryo and hence each testis is progressively pulled down toward the developing scrotum. The testes sit just above the inguinal ring until the last 3 months of pregnancy, at which time they complete their descent through the inguinal canal into the scrotum. After full descent of the testes, the inguinal canal narrows, thereby preventing abdominal contents from herniating into the scrotum. Unlike differentiation of the external and internal genitalia that relies on hCG stimulation of testicular androgen production, testicular descent requires fetal gonadotropins. Disruptions in the fetal hypothalamic–pituitary–testicular axis result in failure of the testes to descend properly (cryptorchidism).

In the female, the folds of the urogenital slit remain open. The posterior aspect of the urogenital sinus forms the **lower two-thirds of the vagina** and the anterior aspect forms the urethra. The lateral genital folds form the **labia minora** and the labioscrotal swellings form the **labia majora**. The **clitoris** forms above the urethra. The gubernaculum that forms between the edge of the Müllerian duct and the ovary becomes secondarily attached to the cornua of the uterus as it differentiates. The gubernaculum in the female becomes the ovarian and round ligaments. Female phenotypic differentiation occurs in the absence of androgen and is not dependent on an ovary.

Exposure to specific androgens beginning in the 5th embryonic (7th menstrual) week of pregnancy is critical to the development of a recognizable newborn male phenotype. Fetuses exposed to endogenous or exogenous DHT at this time will undergo male differentiation, regardless of the genetic or gonadal sex. Lack of androgen activity will result in a female phenotype.

Gross anatomy of the male reproductive tract

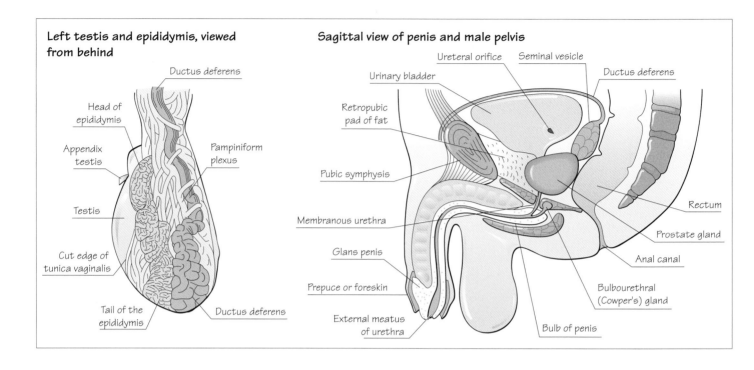

Left testis and epididymis, viewed from behind

- Ductus deferens
- Head of epididymis
- Appendix testis
- Pampiniform plexus
- Testis
- Cut edge of tunica vaginalis
- Tail of the epididymis
- Ductus deferens

Sagittal view of penis and male pelvis

- Ureteral orifice
- Seminal vesicle
- Urinary bladder
- Ductus deferens
- Retropubic pad of fat
- Pubic symphysis
- Rectum
- Membranous urethra
- Prostate gland
- Anal canal
- Glans penis
- Prepuce or foreskin
- Bulbourethral (Cowper's) gland
- External meatus of urethra
- Bulb of penis

Testes and epididymis

The **testes** are a pair of oval, slightly flattened bodies measuring about 4 cm in length and 2.5 cm in diameter. Together with the epididymis, they lie in the scrotum, an extra-abdominal sac just below the penis. The walls of the cavity in which the testes and epididymis reside are known as the **tunica vaginalis**. The tunica vaginalis forms from intra-abdominal peritoneum that migrates into the primitive scrotum during development of the male internal genitalia. After migration of the testis into the scrotum, the channel down which the testis has moved (processus vaginalis) is obliterated.

The **epididymis** is a comma-shaped structure that clasps the postero-lateral margin of the testes. It is formed from an irregularly twisted tube called the duct of the epididymis. The epididymal duct is about 600 cm long. It begins at the top of the testes as the head of the epididymis. After an extraordinarily tortuous course it ends as the tail of the epididymis, then becomes the vas deferens.

The testicular arteries supply blood to the testes and epididymis. These arteries arise from the aorta just below the renal arteries. The testicular arteries end in a dense vascular plexus called the **pampiniform plexus**, which courses just under the tunica vaginalis surrounding the testes. The plexus then drains into the testicular veins. The pampiniform plexus can dissipate heat out of the scrotum by vasodilatation and thereby plays an important role in temperature regulation of the testes. **Like the ovarian veins, the right testicular vein empties into the inferior vena cava, and the left testicular vein into the left renal vein.** Lymphatic drainage of the testes is to the para-aortic nodes.

All the blood and lymph vessels to the testis and epididymis are bundled in a structure known as the **spermatic cord**. This structure also contains the **vas deferens** and any remnants of the processus vaginalis.

The spermatic cord enters the scrotum from the abdomen through the inguinal canal.

The testis is the site of spermatogenesis and sex steroid production in the male. The epididymis is the site of final sperm maturation. The scrotum is basically a specialized dermal pouch that protects the testis and epididymis from physical injury and aids in heat regulation of the testes. Spermatozoa are very heat sensitive. Because the testes and epididymis are outside the body cavity, intratesticular temperature is typically lower than in the abdomen.

Vas (ductus) deferens and seminal vesicles

The vas deferens is a direct continuation of the epididymis. It is a 45-cm-long structure that begins at the lower end of the epididymis and ascends along the posterior aspect of the testis in loose coils. After leaving the back of the testis, the vas deferens traverses the spermatic cord into the abdomen. The vas deferens may be felt as a firm hard cord on the posterior aspect of the spermatic cord as it traverses the scrotum toward the superficial inguinal ring. After crossing into the abdomen, the vas deferens curves medially across the external iliac artery toward the pelvis. From there, it crosses the obturator nerve and vessels and the vesicular vessels. The vas then crosses over the ureter to meet the duct of the seminal vesicle. Together, the vas deferens and the duct of the seminal vesicle form the **ejaculatory duct** that opens into the prostatic portion of the urethra. The ejaculatory duct is short (2.5 cm) and lies very close to its companion contralateral duct as they pass forward through the prostate.

The **seminal vesicles** are a pair of hollow, sacculated structures located at the base of the bladder in front of the rectum. Each vesicle is about 5 cm long and more intimately connected to the bladder than to the rectum. During embryonic development, the seminal vesicles form as diverticula of the vas deferens. The structures share common blood and lymphatic supplies.

The blood supply to the vas deferens and seminal vesicles is mainly from the inferior vesicular artery. The artery accompanies the vas into the scrotum where it anastomoses with the testicular artery. Lymphatic drainage is to the internal and external iliac nodes.

The vas deferens functions in sperm transport. The seminal vesicles produce approximately 50–60% of the volume of the seminal fluid. Important seminal vesicle-derived semen components include fructose and prostaglandins.

Prostate gland

The prostate is a partly glandular, partly muscular organ that surrounds the beginning of the male urethra, firmly affixed by a connective tissue sheath just behind the symphysis pubis. The organ is about $2.5 \times 3.5 \times 4.5$ cm. The median lobe of the prostate, histologically referred to as the transition zone, is wedge-shaped, directly surrounds the urethra and separates it from the ejaculatory ducts. When hypertrophied, the median lobe may obstruct the flow of urine. Median lobe hypertrophy occurs commonly in elderly men.

The anterior prostate is composed mostly of fibromuscular tissue. The glandular tissue of the prostate is situated at the sides of the urethra and immediately posterior to it. This glandular tissue is subdivided into a central and peripheral zone based on embryology (Chapter 7) and histology (Chapter 9). The peripheral zone is much larger than the central zone and composed of about 50 incompletely defined lobules. Each lobule contains minute ducts that empty directly into the urethra just above the ejaculatory ducts.

The blood supply to the prostate gland is variable, but most commonly arises from the common origin of the internal pudendal and inferior gluteal arteries off the internal iliac (hypogastric) arteries. The veins draining the prostate are wide and thin-walled, forming a plexus that communicates with the plexus draining the bladder. Both drain into the internal iliac veins. The prostatic plexus also communicates with the vertebral venous plexuses; therefore, a tumour in the prostate may give rise to secondary growth in the vertebral column. Lymphatic drainage of the prostate follows that of the seminal vesicles and bladder neck into the iliac chain of nodes.

All the muscular tissues in the vas deferens, prostate, prostatic urethra and seminal vesicles are involved in ejaculation. Prostate secretions contribute ~15% of the volume of the seminal fluid. Important prostate-derived components include acid phosphatases, zinc, citrate and proteases that aid in semen liquefaction. Liquefaction enables sperm to escape the very viscous initial ejaculate.

Penis

The penis is composed chiefly of cavernous (erectile) tissue and is traversed by the urethra. The posterior surface of the flaccid penis is nearest the urethra and the opposite, more extensive surface is dorsal.

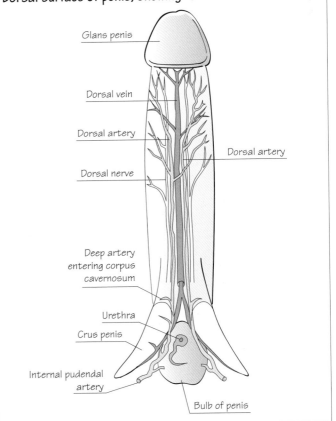

Dorsal surface of penis, showing vessels and nerves

- Glans penis
- Dorsal vein
- Dorsal artery
- Dorsal nerve
- Dorsal artery
- Deep artery entering corpus cavernosum
- Urethra
- Crus penis
- Internal pudendal artery
- Bulb of penis

Most of the erectile tissue of the penis is arranged in three longitudinal columns, the paired **corpora cavernosa** and the single median **corpus spongiosum**. The tip of the penis is called the **glans**. The glans of the penis also contains erectile tissue and is continuous with the corpus spongiosum. The glans is covered with a retractable folded layer of thin skin, called the prepuce or foreskin; it is removed by the operation of circumcision.

The internal pudendal arteries supply blood to the penis, entering the organ on its dorsal surface and penetrating deeply into the erectile tissue of the corpora cavernosa. Veins draining the penis enter the prostatic plexus either directly or through the dorsal vein of the penis. Erection of the penis occurs when the extensive cavernous spaces of the corpora cavernosa and corpus spongiosum fill with blood. Engorgement of the penis inhibits venous return and allows maintenance of erection.

Innervation of the penis is critical for its erection. Penile nerve supply is derived from the pudendal nerve (2nd, 3rd, 4th sacral nerves) and from the pelvic autonomic plexuses. The lymphatic drainage of the penis is into the medial group of superficial inguinal lymph nodes.

The function of the penis is penetration. Penetration of the vagina of the female allows deposition of semen near the uterine cervix.

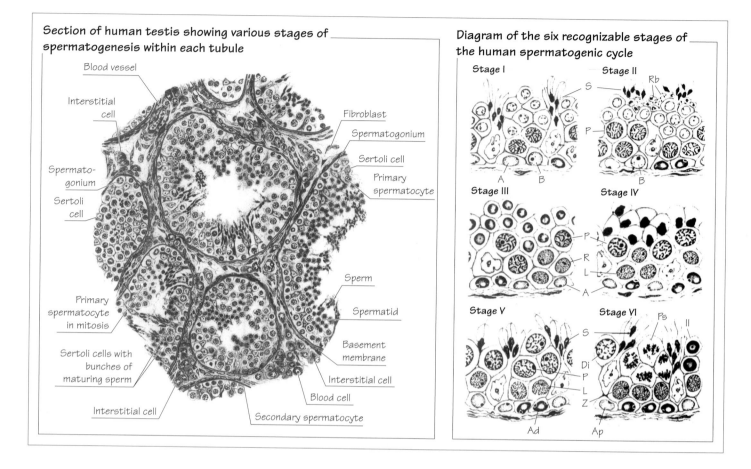

Section of human testis showing various stages of spermatogenesis within each tubule

Blood vessel
Interstitial cell
Spermato-gonium
Sertoli cell
Primary spermatocyte in mitosis
Sertoli cells with bunches of maturing sperm
Interstitial cell

Fibroblast
Spermatogonium
Sertoli cell
Primary spermatocyte
Sperm
Spermatid
Basement membrane
Interstitial cell
Blood cell
Secondary spermatocyte

Diagram of the six recognizable stages of the human spermatogenic cycle

Stage I — S, P, A, B
Stage II — S, Rb, P, B
Stage III — P, R, L, A
Stage IV
Stage V — S, Di, P, L, Z, Ad
Stage VI — Ps, II, Ap

Testes

The testes have two distinct functions, spermatogenesis and androgen production. Spermatogenesis occurs within distinct structures called **seminiferous tubules**. These tubules lie coiled within lobules whose ducts all exit the testes into the epididymis. Androgen production occurs within pockets of specialized cells that lie in the interstitium between the tubules.

The seminiferous tubules are surrounded by a basement membrane. Juxtaposed to the medial side of this basement membrane are the progenitor cells for sperm production. The epithelium containing the developing spermatozoa that line the tubules is known as the **seminiferous epithelium** or **germinal epithelium**. In a cross-section of the testes, spermatocytes within a given tubule are in varying stages of maturation. Mixed among the spermatocytes are **Sertoli cells**. These are the only non-germinal cells in the seminiferous epithelium. Sertoli cells were aptly called 'nurse cells' when first described by Sertoli in 1865. They are responsible for the metabolic and structural support of the developing spermatozoa. All Sertoli cells make contact with the basement membrane at one pole and surround the developing spermatozoa at the other. Sertoli cells have large, complex cytoplasmic 'fingers' that extend around many spermatozoa at one time.

A wide variety of substances that are normally present in the circulation are excluded from the fluid within the seminiferous tubule. This phenomenon is similar to that seen in the brain as the result of the blood–brain barrier. The male reproductive system displays its own **blood–testis barrier**. This barrier allows the testis to be one of very few immune-privileged sites in the human body. While the function of this barrier is incompletely described, its ultrastructural basis is known to be the tight junctions that form between adjacent Sertoli cells. The barriers created by these tight junctions divide the germinal epithelium into basal and luminal compartments. The basement compartment contains the spermatogonia and the luminal compartment, the maturing germinal cells.

Spermatogenesis can be divided into three phases: (i) mitotic proliferation to produce large numbers of cells; (ii) meiotic division to produce genetic diversity; and (iii) maturation. The latter involves extensive cellular morphological remodelling aimed at facilitating sperm transit to, and penetration of, the oocyte in the female tract. Primitive spermatogonial stem cells remain dormant in the testis until puberty. At puberty, they are activated and maintained in rounds of mitoses at the basement membrane of the seminiferous tubule. From this reservoir of self-regenerating stem cells emerge a morphologically distinct group of cells known as A spermatogonia (A). Each one of these A spermatogonia undergoes a limited number of mitotic divisions to form a 'clone' of germ cells. At the next to last mitotic division, the cells are known as B spermatogonia (B) and, after the final division, as primary spermatocytes (Ps). Primary spermatocytes then undergo two meiotic cell divisions. These important divisions halve the number of chromosomes in the daughter cells. Cells undergoing the first of these meiotic divisions have very characteristic differences in their nuclear morphology that has led to a specific nomenclature [resting (R), leptotene (L), zygotene (Z), pachytene and diplotene (Di); Chapter 5]. The first meiotic division produces secondary spermatocytes (II) and the second, early haploid spermatids (S). The spermatids then undergo remarkable cytoplasmic remodelling, during which a tail, mitochondrial midpiece and acrosome all develop. Almost all of the spermatid cytoplasm is expelled. Only a small droplet remains, called the residual body (Rb). It will be removed in the epididymis during the final maturation of the spermatozoon.

Development of the spermatozoa within the seminiferous epithelium is a complex and highly ordered sequence of events in most mammalian species. In humans, the process appears somewhat less orderly, but still follows the general principles found in other species. In each, the number of mitotic divisions the A spermatogonia undergo is fixed. In humans, four mitotic divisions occur. The length of time for an A spermatogonium to develop into a spermatozoon ready to enter the epididymis is also fixed and species-specific. In humans, it takes 64 ± 4 days for this process. As the spermatocytes move through the maturation process, they also move in waves toward the lumen of the seminiferous tubule.

The Sertoli cells enveloping the developing spermatozoa are homologues of the granulosa cells in the ovary. Sertoli cells phagocytose the extruded spermatid cytoplasm. They also function in aromatization of androgen precursors to oestrogen, a product that exerts local feedback regulation on the androgen-producing (Leydig) cells. Sertoli cells also produce androgen-binding proteins.

Leydig cells perform the other major function of the testes–androgen production. The Leydig cells are homologous with the theca cells of the ovary. They produce large amounts of androgen from either circulating cholesterol or cholesterol made internally within their own smooth endoplasmic reticulum. Leydig cells are very large and, consistent with their intracellular activities, appear foamy by standard histological assessment.

The most easily damaged cells in the testis are the spermatogonia. Irradiation, excessive alcohol intake, dietary deficiencies and local inflammation can rapidly induce degenerative changes in these cells. Excess heat also induces extensive spermatogonial cell degeneration but does not affect the length of the spermatogenic cycle.

Epididymis and vas (ductus) deferens

The ducts forming the epididymis and vas deferens have muscular coats composed of an inner layer of circularly directed fibres and an outer layer of longitudinally directed fibres. The muscle component of these structures is responsible for peristalsis that moves the spermatozoa along the ducts. The ducts are lined with a mixture of secretory and ciliated cells. The former aid in the generation of intratubal fluids; the latter assist in directed transit of intratubal fluids and cellular components.

Seminal vesicles

The alveoli of the seminal vesicles are lined with a pseudostratified epithelium whose cells contain numerous granules and clumps of yellow pigment. Some of the epithelial cells have flagella. The secretion of the seminal vesicles is a yellowish, viscous liquid containing globulin and fructose. This secretion provides the majority of the ejaculate volume.

Prostate gland

The tubuloalveolar glands of the prostate are lined with an epithelium that is highly responsive to androgens. The acini of the central glandular zone that surrounds the ejaculatory ducts are large and irregular. By contrast, the acini of the peripheral glandular zone are small and regular. These striking differences in glandular architecture, along with the observation that several unique enzymes present in the seminal vesicles are present in the central but not the peripheral glandular zone, suggests different embryological tissue origins for these two parts of the prostate (Chapter 7). The epithelium of the prostatic tubuloalveolar glands produces the acid phosphatase and citric acid normally found in semen.

Penis

The erectile tissue of the penis is a vast, sponge-like system of irregular vascular spaces fed by the afferent arterioles and drained by the efferent venules. A pair of cylindrical bodies, the corpora cavernosa, are surrounded by a thick fibrous membrane called the tunica albuginea and separated by an incomplete fibrous septum. The veins draining the cavernous bodies lie just beneath the tunica. The interior of the cavernous bodies contains many partitions called trabeculae. Trabeculae are comprised of elastic fibres and smooth muscle embedded within thick bundles of collagen and covered by endothelial cells.

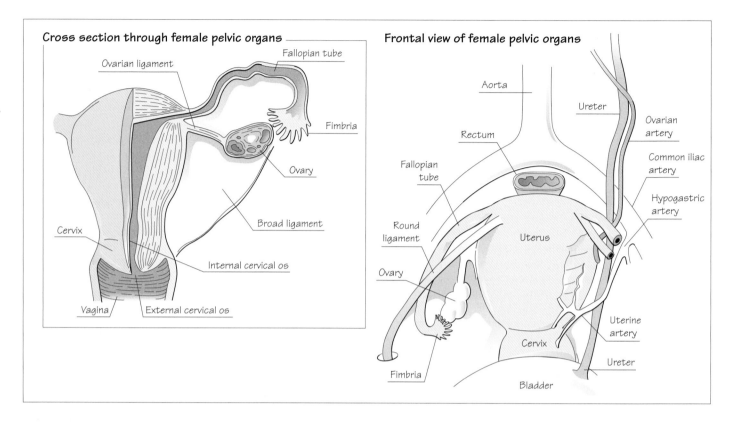

Cross section through female pelvic organs — Ovarian ligament, Fallopian tube, Fimbria, Ovary, Broad ligament, Cervix, Internal cervical os, Vagina, External cervical os

Frontal view of female pelvic organs — Aorta, Ureter, Ovarian artery, Common iliac artery, Hypogastric artery, Rectum, Fallopian tube, Round ligament, Uterus, Ovary, Uterine artery, Cervix, Ureter, Fimbria, Bladder

Ovaries

The ovaries are two small oval structures, each about $2 \times 4 \times 1.5$ cm, lying deep within the female pelvis just lateral to, and behind, the uterus. They are loosely attached to the uterus by a connective tissue band. To the practitioner performing a bimanual exam, they feel much like almonds sliding between the examiner's palpating fingers. After menopause, they may not be palpable at all.

The ovarian artery arises from the aorta just below the renal artery and is the ovary's major source of blood. The ovarian artery courses through the retroperitoneal space of the abdomen in close proximity to the ureter. Blood draining the ovaries traverses the ovarian veins. **The ovarian veins empty into the vena cava on the right and the renal vein on the left**. This anatomical difference in venous drainage is important: the more lateral position of the left ovarian vein makes it more susceptible to obstruction and thrombus formation, especially in pregnancy. The lymphatic drainage of the ovary feeds into the lumbar (para-aortic) nodes.

The functions of the ovaries are to produce mature ova for fertilization and to generate large quantities of steroid hormones.

Fallopian tubes

These are bilateral hollow structures that attach to the uterus at each cornua (corner). The Fallopian tube is divided anatomically and functionally into three sections, the **cornua**, **isthmus** and **fimbria**. The cornual section is contained within the muscular wall of the uterus and provides a stable, strong connection with this organ. Fertilization occurs in the long, narrow, pencil-like portion called the isthmus. The fimbriated, or fluted, end of the tube is the most distal portion. The fimbria are finger-like distal projections of the Fallopian tubes. They display continual sweeping-like activity and are known to reach into the cul-de-sac of the female pelvis to retrieve ovulated eggs that fall behind the uterus.

The fimbria of the Fallopian tube are not enclosed within the parietal peritoneum of the broad ligament and hence communicate with the abdominal cavity. This anatomic connection creates the potential for foreign matter that enters the vagina (i.e. bacteria, sperm and chemicals) to gain access to the abdominal cavity by traversing the cervical canal, uterus and Fallopian tube. This has important implications for exposure of the intraperitoneal cavity to carcinogens and for intraperitoneal spread of infections ascending through the reproductive tract (Chapters 41 and 45–7, respectively).

The blood supply to the Fallopian tube is largely through the ovarian vessels, although anastomoses with ascending branches of the uterine artery occur within the broad ligament. The lymphatic drainage of the tube follows that of the ovary into the para-aortic nodes.

The functions of the Fallopian tube include transporting sperm and eggs to the site of fertilization within the tube and returning the fertilized zygote to the uterine cavity for implantation.

Together with the ovaries, the Fallopian tubes are covered with a layer of parietal peritoneum known as the **broad ligament**. This forms a double-thickness draping structure that is bounded superiorly by the round ligament of the uterus. The broad ligament connects the uterus, Fallopian tubes and ovaries to the pelvic sidewall just lateral to these structures. It contains important blood vessels, including the uterine arteries and veins.

Uterus

The uterus is a single, pear-shaped, muscular structure that sits between the bladder and rectum in the female pelvis. A mature uterus weighs 30–40 g in a woman who has never delivered a baby and 75–100 g in one who has. It is anchored in the pelvis by three sets of connective tissue ligaments: the **round**, **cardinal** and **uterosacral ligaments**. The round ligaments attach to the cornua of the uterus anterior to the insertion of the Fallopian tubes. These distinct cord-like structures traverse the pelvis, enter the inguinal rings bilaterally and attach firmly to the osteum of the pelvic bone. They provide some stability to the upper pole of the uterus but are not essential. The cardinal ligaments connect the uterus to the anterior abdominal wall at the level of the cervix. The uterosacral ligaments attach to the uterus posteriorly at the level of the cervix and connect to the sacral bones. The cardinal and uterosacral ligaments provide significant support to the female pelvic floor. Damage to these ligaments, including undue stretching from childbirth, can allow prolapse of the uterus and pelvic floor into the vagina or even through the vagina and onto the vulva.

The uterus is divided into three anatomically and functionally distinct areas, the **cervix**, the **lower uterine segment** and the uterine **corpus**. The cervix is composed largely of firm connective tissue and is typically about 4 cm long. About 2 cm of this protrudes into the vagina; the remainder is intraperitoneal. The cervix opens into the uterus via the internal os and into the vagina via the external os. The lower uterine segment includes the lower third of the uterus. The muscle of the lower segment draws the dilating cervix up and thins in labour. The corpus, the largest segment of the uterus, is composed of thick muscle. The very top of the uterus between the Fallopian tubes is called the **fundus**, a term sometimes used to refer to the entire corpus of the uterus.

The blood supply of the uterus is complex. The fundus is supplied by vessels stemming from the ovarian arteries while the corpus, lower segment and cervix are supplied by the uterine arteries. The uterine artery is the largest branch of the anterior division of the internal iliac artery (also known as the hypogastric artery). The uterine artery travels from the pelvic sidewall to the uterus at the level of the internal cervical os and the cardinal and uterosacral ligaments. In doing so, the uterine artery crosses over the ureter, which is coursing directly from the kidney toward the bladder. This anatomical relationship must be kept in mind during all pelvic surgery involving the uterus and its blood supply. Failure to remember that 'water runs under the bridge' has caused many an avoidable ureteral injury.

The lymphatic drainage of the uterus follows its blood supply. The fundus and upper part of the body drain, like the ovaries, to lymph nodes in the para-aortic chain. The lower part of the body of the uterus and the cervix drain into nodes located along the internal and external iliac vessels.

The function of the uterus is to provide support for the growing fetus during pregnancy.

Vagina

A tubular structure that spans the distance between its opening at the introitus of the perineum and the cervix. Its surface is covered with a compliant, rugated-appearing epithelium. The upper two-thirds is most correctly considered part of the internal genitalia because of its embryological relationship with the uterus. The hymen, which may remain as a thin transverse membrane through puberty or first sexual intercourse, is seen as an irregular circle of tissue at the opening of the vagina onto the vulva.

The function of the vagina is to hold the penis during intercourse and to serve as a temporary receptacle for semen.

Vulva

The external female genitalia are collectively known as the vulva. The vulva comprises the **lower one-third of the vagina**, the **clitoris** and the **labia**. The labia majora are the largest structures of the external female genitalia and surround the other organs, ending in the mons pubis. The mons pubis is a large fatty prominence that lies over the pubic symphysis. The mons and the labia majora are the only visible parts of the female external genitalia. One must part the labia majora to see the labia minora, clitoris and urethral opening. There are **numerous mucus-secreting glands** lining the vaginal opening. The largest and most important of these extend posterolaterally towards the buttocks and are called the Bartholin's glands.

The internal pudendal artery supplies blood to the vulva; it derives from the posterior division of the internal iliac artery. The lymph drainage is into the inguinal nodes.

The clitoris is the homologue of the penis and the organ of sexual arousal in the female.

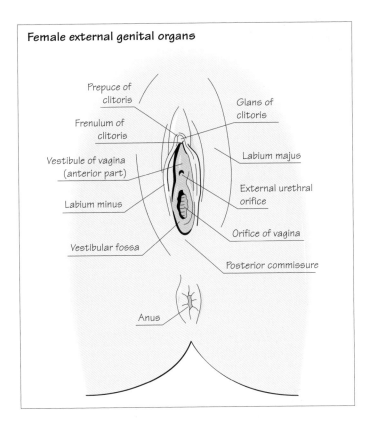

Female external genital organs

- Prepuce of clitoris
- Frenulum of clitoris
- Vestibule of vagina (anterior part)
- Labium minus
- Vestibular fossa
- Glans of clitoris
- Labium majus
- External urethral orifice
- Orifice of vagina
- Posterior commissure
- Anus

Cross section of the human ovary

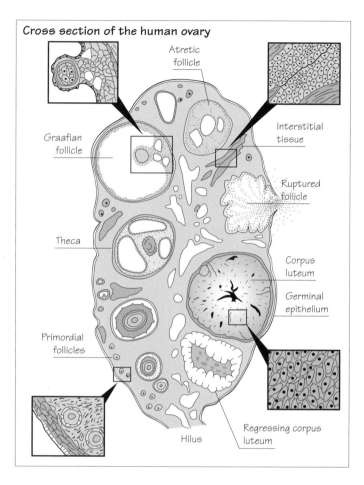

Cross section of the human ovary: Atretic follicle, Graafian follicle, Interstitial tissue, Ruptured follicle, Theca, Corpus luteum, Germinal epithelium, Primordial follicles, Regressing corpus luteum, Hilus

surrounding granulosa cells from flat to cuboidal; (iii) an increase in granulosa cell number; and (iv) the appearance of a **zona pellucida** around the oocyte. The zona pellucida is a sphere of gelatinous protein matrix immediately surrounding the oocyte. Once growth of the granulosa cells has produced 3–4 layers of cells, fluid begins to accumulate between the cells. This fluid resembles blood plasma and contains high concentrations of several protein and steroid hormones. When this follicular fluid accumulates around the oocyte, the follicle is known as a **Graffian follicle** and is approaching ovulation. Although as many as 20 follicles begin to mature in each wave of recruitment, typically only one successfully ovulates.

Ovulation involves expulsion of the egg through a thinned-out area known as the stigma. Stigmata can be seen with the naked eye as 'blisters' on the surface of the ovary. After the oocyte is released, the follicle collapses and the granulosa cells proliferate to fill the space left by the released oocyte and its associated follicular fluid. They undergo a remarkable transformation into plump, endocrinologically active cells known as lutein cells. These lutein cells produce a yellow pigment and the structure containing these cells is appropriately called the **corpus luteum**, or yellow body. During corpus luteum formation, blood vessels penetrate the follicular basement membrane.

Fallopian tube

The lumen of the Fallopian tube is covered by a columnar epithelium with long **cilia** on the surface of many of the cells. The cilia are constantly beating toward the uterus, a function that facilitates movement of the non-motile zygote toward the uterine cavity for implantation. When the cilia are injured or incapable of movement, an embryo may inappropriately implant within the Fallopian tube itself (**ectopic pregnancy**).

Uterus

The vast majority of the uterine wall is composed of smooth muscle, called **myometrium**. The smooth muscle cells of the myometrium (myocytes) are attached by gap junctions, allowing rapid communication among neighbouring cells and coordinated movement of the entire muscle mass. The uterus must be capable of enormous growth during pregnancy. This is accomplished by hypertrophy of the myocytes and by recruitment of new myocytes from stem cells residing within the myometrial connective tissue.

The cavity of the uterus is lined by a glandular epithelium, the **endometrium**. The endometrium is both an endocrine target organ and a gland. Under the influence of cyclic hormone production by the ovary, the endometrium undergoes striking microscopic changes in its glandular structure and function. During the preovulatory phase of the menstrual cycle, the epithelial cells on the surface of the endometrium proliferate profusely under the influence of oestrogen. The glands proliferate and elongate deep into the subepithelial layer known as the endometrial stroma. Small muscular arteries known as **spiral arteries** grow inward from the basal layer of the endometrium between the elongating glands. The hallmark of the **proliferative endometrium** is frequent mitoses in the epithelium. Immediately prior to ovulation, the endometrial glands are maximally elongated and markedly coiled.

With ovulation, the hormonal environment within the uterus changes from oestrogen-dominant to progesterone-dominant. In response to this

Ovary

The ovary has two distinct functions, germ cell production and steroid hormone biosynthesis. Germ cell support occurs in microscopic structures known as ovarian follicles. Resting follicles each contain a primitive or **primordial oocyte** surrounded by a single layer of cells, the **granulosa cells**. Surrounding the granulosa cells are a collar of cells known as **theca cells**. Theca cells produce androgens that are then converted to oestrogens by the granulosa cells (Chapter 3). Steroid hormones produced by the ovary act within the follicle to support the developing oocyte and outside the ovary on target tissues.

The human ovary contains about 2 million oocytes at birth but only 100 000 at puberty. The number of oocytes continues to decrease throughout a woman's reproductive life span. This decrease occurs because mitosis of the primitive oogonia stops midway through fetal life and does not resume. At the time mitosis stops, the newly formed oocytes enter into the prophase of the first meiotic division. They will remain in meiotic prophase until either they are stimulated to mature for ovulation or they degenerate in a process called **atresia**.

The primordial follicles are scattered just beneath the connective tissue capsule covering the ovary. This superficial position permits ovulation into the abdominal cavity. The earliest signs of follicular growth are: (i) an increase in size of the oocyte; (ii) a change in the shape of the

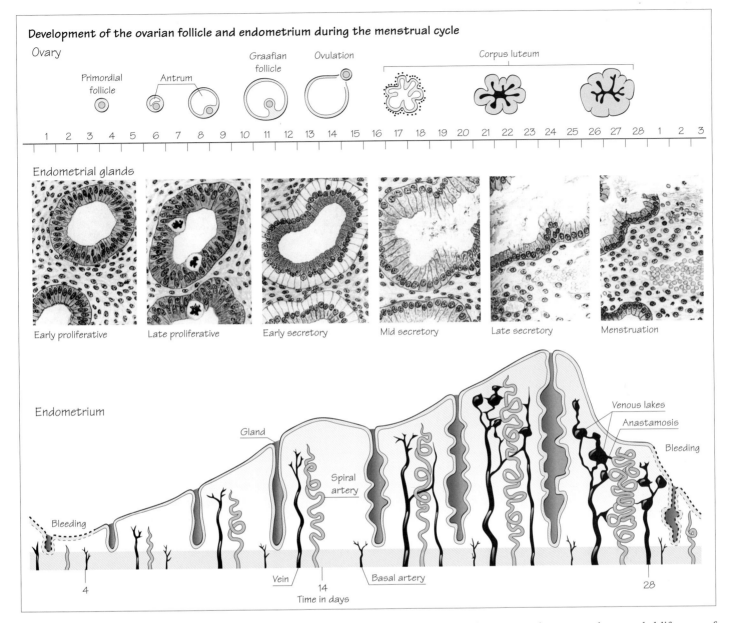

Development of the ovarian follicle and endometrium during the menstrual cycle

Ovary

Primordial follicle | Antrum | Graafian follicle | Ovulation | Corpus luteum

1 2 3 4 5 6 7 8 9 10 11 12 13 14 15 16 17 18 19 20 21 22 23 24 25 26 27 28 1 2 3

Endometrial glands

Early proliferative | Late proliferative | Early secretory | Mid secretory | Late secretory | Menstruation

Endometrium

Gland

Spiral artery

Venous lakes
Anastamosis
Bleeding

Bleeding

Vein | 14 | Basal artery | 28

4

Time in days

change, mitosis ceases in the glandular epithelium and the cells form a single columnar layer within the glands. Within 2 days of ovulation, small subnuclear vacuoles form in the cytoplasm of the columnar cells. These secretory vacuoles are rich in glycogen and lipid and, by 4 days after ovulation, they migrate to the luminal side of the cells. Over the next 2 days, the vacuoles discharge their contents into the glandular lumens, leaving the borders of the glandular cells frayed in appearance. This activity is the basis for the term **secretory endometrium**, which is used to describe the postovulatory endometrial changes.

Concurrent with these glandular changes are marked alterations in the endometrial stromal cells. With ovulation, stromal cells enlarge and acquire a foamy appearance indicative of increased metabolism. These cells become very eosinophilic and are known as decidual cells. **Decidualization** of the endometrium begins around the elongated and coiled spiral arteries. Decidualization then spreads under the surface epithelium and glands by 10 days after ovulation.

If implantation does not occur in a given menstrual cycle, progesterone production by the corpus luteum stops by day 13–14 postovulation. The endometrium undergoes ischemic necrosis and sloughs off, shed as

menstrual debris. If pregnancy does occur, the extended life span of the corpus luteum will prolong its progesterone production and decidualization of the stroma will continue. The endometrial stroma is an important source of several peptides in pregnancy, including prolactin, insulin-like growth factor binding protein 1 (IGFBP-1) and parathyroid hormone-related peptide (PTHrP).

The hormone-driven histological changes in the endometrium are so predictable that they can be used to document ovulation and its timing.

Cervix and vagina

The cervix is composed largely of connective tissue. This is covered by a layer of mucus-secreting **glandular epithelium** inside the cervical canal (endocervix) and a stratified **squamous epithelium** on the portion of the cervix visible within the vagina (ectocervix). The transition between the glandular and squamous epithelium is known as the transformation zone. The **transformation zone** typically occurs just inside the external os of the cervix. The zone is important in that it is a common site of dysplastic changes that can become malignant. The vagina is covered with squamous epithelium.

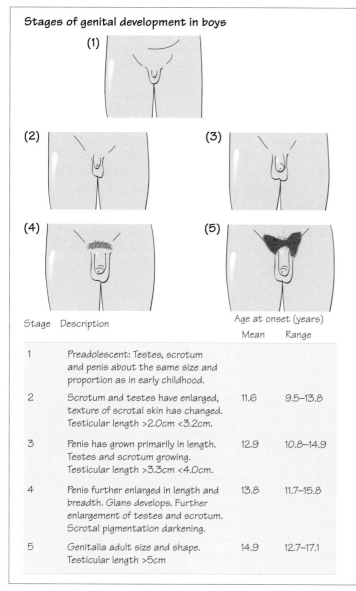

Stages of genital development in boys

Stage	Description	Age at onset (years)	
		Mean	Range
1	Preadolescent: Testes, scrotum and penis about the same size and proportion as in early childhood.		
2	Scrotum and testes have enlarged, texture of scrotal skin has changed. Testicular length >2.0cm <3.2cm.	11.6	9.5–13.8
3	Penis has grown primarily in length. Testes and scrotum growing. Testicular length >3.3cm <4.0cm.	12.9	10.8–14.9
4	Penis further enlarged in length and breadth. Glans develops. Further enlargement of testes and scrotum. Scrotal pigmentation darkening.	13.8	11.7–15.8
5	Genitalia adult size and shape. Testicular length >5cm	14.9	12.7–17.1

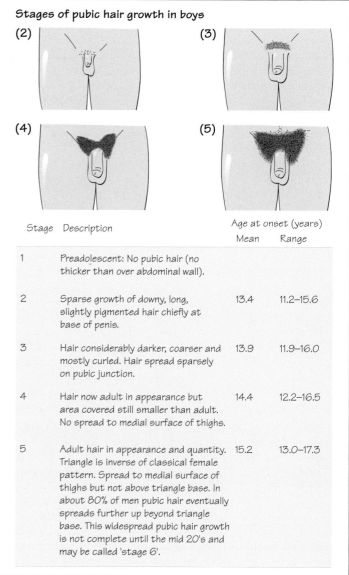

Stages of pubic hair growth in boys

Stage	Description	Age at onset (years)	
		Mean	Range
1	Preadolescent: No pubic hair (no thicker than over abdominal wall).		
2	Sparse growth of downy, long, slightly pigmented hair chiefly at base of penis.	13.4	11.2–15.6
3	Hair considerably darker, coarser and mostly curled. Hair spread sparsely on pubic junction.	13.9	11.9–16.0
4	Hair now adult in appearance but area covered still smaller than adult. No spread to medial surface of thighs.	14.4	12.2–16.5
5	Adult hair in appearance and quantity. Triangle is inverse of classical female pattern. Spread to medial surface of thighs but not above triangle base. In about 80% of men pubic hair eventually spreads further up beyond triangle base. This widespread pubic hair growth is not complete until the mid 20's and may be called 'stage 6'.	15.2	13.0–17.3

Puberty is the process by which the immature individual will acquire the physical and behavioural attributes that allow him or her to reproduce. In males, puberty is largely the response of the body to widespread actions of androgens. These are secreted by the newly awakened testes, under the influence of gonadotropins secreted by the anterior pituitary. While the progression of pubertal changes is predictable, the age of their onset differs dramatically in different areas of the world and even among children of different ethnic backgrounds within a particular region. Economic disparities may also be reflected in the age of onset.

Physical changes of puberty

In North America and Europe, puberty visibly begins with testes enlargement between ages 9 and 14. Secondary sexual characteristics progressively appear over the ensuing 2–2.5 years, and facial hair, the last to appear, will not be fully mature until ages 20–25.

The physical changes of puberty in boys have been divided into five stages using a system developed by Marshall and Tanner, who examined groups of English boys as they went through sexual maturation. They then classified the relative and absolute changes in the sexual characteristics of the participants. Although they did not regard their findings as universal, their system has been widely used to describe the timing and progression of typical pubertal changes. Their descriptions must be recognized as specific to the demographics of their study population and to the years covered by the study. Patterns persist, but the characteristics and timing of these changes are affected by race, nutrition, and other genetic and environmental factors.

Adrenarche

This describes the contribution of the adrenal gland to puberty. It is characterized by an increase in adrenal synthesis and secretion of the relatively weak androgens: androstenedione, dehydroepiandrosterone (DHEA), and dehydroepiandrosterone sulfate (DHEA-S). Although the adrenal gland contributes only 5% of the total circulating androgen pool in boys, these adrenal androgens are responsible for initiating axillary and pubic hair growth. They are converted in the periphery to the more potent androgens: testosterone and dihydrotestosterone (DHT). Testosterone and DHT then stimulate pubic and axillary hair growth as well as growth of, and secretion by, the axillary sebaceous glands. Axillary and pubic hair typically appear in parallel with increasing testicular size and visibly mark the onset of puberty.

The exact trigger for adrenarche is unknown. The best evidence indicates it is an intrinsic, programmed event within the adrenal gland independent of adrenocorticotropic hormone (ACTH). Adrenarche is distinct from pubarche and either may occur in the absence of its counterpart.

Testicular maturation

Maturation of the testes at puberty involves initiation of androgen production by the Leydig cells, growth of the seminiferous tubules and initiation of spermatogenesis. All three events are controlled by the gonadotropins: follicle-stimulating hormone (FSH) and luteinizing hormone (LH).

Throughout childhood, FSH and LH concentrations in both the pituitary gland and plasma are low. Pulse amplitude and frequency of both hormones are also low, suggesting that the gonadotropin-releasing hormone (GnRH) pulse generator is cycling slowly. This characteristic of the gonadotropin–pituitary axis has been called the juvenile pause. About a year before testicular enlargement occurs, the release of pulsatile FSH and LH begins to increase in both amplitude and concentration. When this begins, it is most notable during sleep. This marked diurnal rhythm in FSH and LH secretion is the first endocrinological manifestation of puberty. While these diurnal variations may be striking during early and mid-puberty, they are almost obliterated by the end of puberty.

The initiation of puberty is thought to reflect the release of the hypothalamic GnRH pulse generator from CNS inhibition. The site and exact mechanism of this inhibitory release are not known. While much evidence indicates that the source of the trigger also resides in the CNS, there is growing interest in the role of leptin, a hormone produced by fat cells, in the initiation and progression of puberty. Leptin has been shown to be one of the many factors that influence the maturation of the GnRH pulse generator. Individuals who lack the hypothalamic GnRH pulse generator do not undergo puberty (Kallman syndrome, see Chapter 29) and tumours or surgery in the region of the median basal hypothalamus can be associated with delayed or absent puberty.

The increase in size of the testes with onset of puberty is largely the result of increasing mass of the seminiferous tubules and initiation of spermatogenesis. Leydig cell stimulation results in a 10-fold increase in testosterone production over the course of puberty but accounts for only a small proportion of the change in testicular size. The Leydig cells occupy less than 10% of the total testicular mass.

Secondary sexual characteristics

Testosterone and its metabolites cause the following somatic changes in pubertal boys:
- Increased laryngeal size.
- Deepening of the voice.
- Increased bone mass.
- Increased mass and strength of skeletal muscle.
- Thickened skin.
- Increased and thickened hair on the trunk, pubis, axillae and face.

Somatic growth

Somatic growth at puberty is the result of a complex interaction between gonadal sex steroids, growth hormone (GH) and insulin-like growth factor I (IGF-I). Insulin and thyroxine are also necessary for optimal growth. The absence of GH, IGF-I or IGF-I receptor will lead to somatic dwarfism, even in the presence of normal plasma sex steroid concentrations.

Concomitant with the changes in the pulse frequency of LH that signal the beginning of puberty is a change in the amplitude of GH secretion. This appears to be the result of oestrogen stimulation in both boys and girls. In boys, while the increase in GH can be initiated and maintained by testosterone, it does not occur with the administration of DHT. Further, GH secretion in the presence of testosterone can be blocked by the administration of tamoxifen, which blocks the oestrogen receptor. In contrast, even miniscule doses of oestrogen substantially increase GH concentrations. These findings suggest that the effect of testosterone on bone growth is indirect and probably secondary to aromatization of testosterone to oestradiol. This is in stark contrast to the action of testosterone on muscle, where androgens act directly to increase muscle mass.

Bone growth occurs when testosterone, aromatized to oestradiol, increases GH levels. This causes a parallel rise in IGF-I, a potent anabolic hormone that mediates many metabolic actions of GH, including trabecular bone formation. Normally GH stimulates IGF-I synthesis, and IGF-I suppresses GH release in a negative feedback loop. At puberty, however, GH continues to rise despite high levels of circulating IGF-I. This allows for maximum linear bone growth during puberty. Outside of puberty, this combination of an increase in both GH and IGF-I is seen only in acromegaly, a disease state characterized by autonomous GH secretion. Peak growth velocity in boys occurs when plasma testosterone levels reach 50% of adult male levels, and growth will continue until epiphyseal fusion occurs in the long bones. The sex steroids (perhaps via oestrogen activity) are responsible for epiphyseal closure, which occurs at a median age of 21 in young men.

The determinants of final adult height are many and include genetic predisposition, body mass index at the onset of puberty, nutrition and length of puberty. Genetic determinants of bone growth appear to be carried on the distal short arm of the X chromosome. This locus does not appear to undergo X inactivation. Therefore, this locus, and any homologous loci on the Y chromosome, will direct final adult height. The effects of this genetic control pattern are particularly notable among men with the sex chromosome disorder called Klinefelter syndrome; they have a 47XXY karyotype and are unusually tall, presumably because of the double dose of X-linked stature determinants.

Higher body mass indices in late childhood affect final height in both boys and girls. Children with increased body fat tend to enter puberty earlier. They begin their growth spurt after a shorter period of prepubertal growth and hence may not reach the full genetically predetermined adult height. Boys enter puberty later than girls and so have a longer period of prepubertal growth. Boys also experience a greater peak linear growth velocity during adolescence than girls. For both reasons, men tend to be taller than women.

Androgens have a direct anabolic effect on muscle mass. The increase in androgen secretion during puberty increases muscle mass in both boys and girls. Reflecting the higher levels of circulating androgens, this effect is more dramatic in boys.

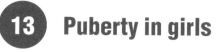

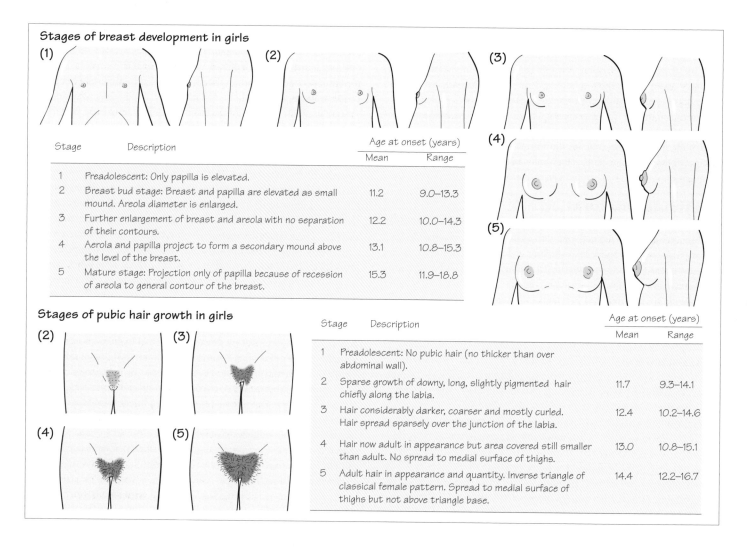

Stages of breast development in girls

(1) (2) (3) (4) (5)

Stage	Description	Age at onset (years)	
		Mean	Range
1	Preadolescent: Only papilla is elevated.		
2	Breast bud stage: Breast and papilla are elevated as small mound. Areola diameter is enlarged.	11.2	9.0–13.3
3	Further enlargement of breast and areola with no separation of their contours.	12.2	10.0–14.3
4	Aerola and papilla project to form a secondary mound above the level of the breast.	13.1	10.8–15.3
5	Mature stage: Projection only of papilla because of recession of areola to general contour of the breast.	15.3	11.9–18.8

Stages of pubic hair growth in girls

(2) (3) (4) (5)

Stage	Description	Age at onset (years)	
		Mean	Range
1	Preadolescent: No pubic hair (no thicker than over abdominal wall).		
2	Sparse growth of downy, long, slightly pigmented hair chiefly along the labia.	11.7	9.3–14.1
3	Hair considerably darker, coarser and mostly curled. Hair spread sparsely over the junction of the labia.	12.4	10.2–14.6
4	Hair now adult in appearance but area covered still smaller than adult. No spread to medial surface of thighs.	13.0	10.8–15.1
5	Adult hair in appearance and quantity. Inverse triangle of classical female pattern. Spread to medial surface of thighs but not above triangle base.	14.4	12.2–16.7

Puberty is the process by which the immature individual will acquire the physical and behavioural attributes that allow him or her to reproduce. In girls, puberty is largely the response of the body to the widespread actions of oestrogens, secreted by the newly awakened ovary under the influence of gonadotropins secreted by the anterior pituitary. While the progression of pubertal changes is predictable, age of onset differs dramatically in different areas of the world and even among children of different ethnic backgrounds within a particular region. Economic disparities may also be reflected in the age of pubertal onset.

Physical changes of puberty

In North American and European girls, puberty visibly begins with breast development between the ages of 8 and 10. Other secondary sexual characteristics appear over the ensuing 2.5 years. Puberty culminates with onset of menstruation. The average age of menarche in Caucasian girls is 12.8 ± 1.2 years and, on average, 4–8 months earlier in African-American girls.

The physical changes of puberty in girls have been divided into five stages using a system developed by Marshall and Tanner, who examined groups of English girls as they went through sexual maturation.

They then classified the relative and absolute changes in the sexual characteristics of the participants. Although they did not regard their findings as universal, their system has been widely used to describe the timing and progression of typical pubertal changes. Their descriptions must be recognized as specific to the demographics of their study population and to the years covered by the study. Patterns persist, but the characteristics and timing of these changes are affected by race, nutrition, and other genetic and environmental factors.

Adrenarche

This describes the contribution of the adrenal gland to puberty in both girls and boys. It is a developmentally programmed increase in adrenal synthesis and secretion of the weak androgens: androstenedione, dehydroepiandrosterone (DHEA) and dehydroepiandrosterone sulfate (DHEA-S). Adrenarche begins at about ages 6–8 years in girls. Secretion of weak adrenal androgens precedes the visible onset of puberty by about 2 years. DHEA and DHEA-S are responsible for initiating growth of pubic and axillary hair as well as growth of and secretion by axillary sebaceous glands. Axillary and pubic hair appear in parallel with the beginning of breast development and visibly mark the onset of puberty in girls.

The exact trigger for adrenarche is not known. It is independent of ACTH release, gonadotropin release, and ovarian function, and appears to be an intrinsic, programmed event within the adrenal gland. Adrenarche is distinct from the other events of puberty (pubarche) and either may occur in the absence of its counterpart.

Menarche

The term used to describe the onset of menstrual cycles. It is the culmination of a complex sequence of events that involves maturation of the hypothalamic–pituitary–ovarian (H–P–O) axis to produce both mature ova and an endometrium that can support a zygote if fertilization should occur. The three stages of maturation of the H–P–O axis include: (i) an increase in the release of follicle-stimulating hormone (FSH) and luteinizing hormone (LH) from the pituitary gland; (ii) ovarian recognition of, and response to these gonadotropins, allowing production of ovarian steroids (oestrogen and progesterone); (iii) establishment of positive feedback regulation of the hypothalamus and pituitary gland by oestrogens. The combination of these maturational events permits ovulation.

Throughout childhood, FSH and LH concentrations within the pituitary gland and plasma of boys and girls are low. As described in Chapter 12, the pulse amplitude and frequency of FSH and LH release are also low, suggesting the gonadotropin-releasing hormone (GnRH) pulse generator is cycling slowly. This characteristic pattern has been called the juvenile pause. The first endocrinological manifestation of puberty is an increase in FSH and LH pulse amplitude. At its initiation, this increase is most notable during sleep, although the diurnal sleep–awake difference in FSH and LH secretion is almost obliterated by the end of puberty.

The initiation of puberty remains incompletely understood. Still, most agree it must be related to a release of the hypothalamic GnRH pulse generator from CNS inhibition.

There has been much interest in the observation that the age of menarche decreased by 2–3 months per decade during the 150 years preceding World War II and then stabilized over the next 50 years. A decrease was again noted in recent studies, thought to represent the influence of optimal nutrition. Onset of menarche is closely related to attainment of a crucial percentage of body fat. Two metabolic signals have been recently identified that can act centrally and may be causal in pubertal events: insulin-like growth factor I (IGF-I) and leptin. Serum IGF-I levels increase during childhood and peak at puberty: the increase parallels that of DHEA-S, the marker of adrenarche. Leptin, a hormone signalling satiety, inhibits neuropeptide Y (NPY). NPY is a mediator of food intake, but also controls GnRH neuronal activity in the hypothalamus. Serum leptin levels increase in boys and girls just before onset of puberty. **Rising leptin levels inhibit NPY. This, in turn, releases GnRH from its prepubertal inhibition.** Leptin levels continue to rise throughout puberty among healthy females, but fall fairly rapidly after pubertal initiation in males.

Maturation of the ovary at puberty allows initiation of oestrogen production by the granulosa cells surrounding the ova. Waves of granulosa cells undergo development and subsequent atresia as puberty progresses. Ova begin to mature under the influence of ovarian oestrogen produced by these granulosa cells. In addition to oocyte maturation, oestrogen from the granulosa cells will regulate production of gonadotropins by the pituitary gland. With complete maturation of the H–P–O axis, this oestrogen will drive maturation of a dominant ovarian follicle, culminating in ovulation. With ovulation of the first ovum, the collapsing ovarian follicle reconfigures itself as a corpus luteum and begins to produce progesterone. The endometrium responds to oestrogen by proliferating and to progesterone by converting to a secretory tissue

capable of supporting embryo implantation. In the first years after menarche many menstrual cycles will be anovulatory, reflecting the incomplete maturation of the hypothalamic positive feedback response to ovarian oestrogen. The menstrual bleeding patterns often encountered soon after menarche represent continuous exposure of the endometrium to oestrogen and sloughing of proliferative or hyperplastic endometrium. Because no corpus luteum forms in the absence of ovulation, the endometrium cannot exhibit the progesterone effect that makes menstruation a self-limited phenomenon. This anovulatory bleeding can be very unpredictable and quite heavy. By 5 years after onset of menarche, 90% of girls have regular, ovulatory menstrual cycles.

Breast development (thelarche)

The mammary gland, or breast, is an ectodermal derivative. The breast tissues are remarkably sensitive to hormones. Hormonal effects are most notable during embryonic development and after puberty. The basic structure of the breast is common to all mammals although there exist wide variations in the number of mammary glands, their size, location and shape. Each mammary gland comprises lobulated masses of glandular tissue. Glandular tissues are embedded in adipose tissue and separated by fibrous connective tissues. Each of the lobes contains lobules of alveoli, blood vessels and lactiferous ducts. See Chapter 23 for a more detailed description of the structure and function of the human breast.

At birth, the breasts consist almost entirely of lactiferous ducts with few, if any, alveoli. These rudimentary mammary glands are capable of a small degree of secretory function (witch's milk) within a few days of birth. Breast secretion in the neonatal period occurs in response to the high prolactin levels in the newborn infant following prior exposure of the fetal breast to high concentrations of placental oestrogen during gestation. Once the placental oestrogens are cleared from the neonatal circulation, the breast enters a quiescent phase until puberty.

With the onset of puberty, ovarian oestrogens induce growth of the lactiferous duct system. The ducts branch as they grow and their ends begin to form into small, solid spheroidal masses of cells. These structures will form the lobular alveoli. The breast and alveoli enlarge. With menarche, cyclic oestrogen and progesterone secretion begin and an additional phase of ductal and rudimentary lobular growth will occur. Adrenal corticosteroids further enhance duct development. The breasts continue to increase in size for some time after menarche due to deposition of fat and additional connective tissue. Final differentiation and growth of the breast will not occur until pregnancy.

Secondary sexual characteristics

Ovarian oestrogens also produce the following changes in pubertal girls:
- Pubic hair.
- Keratinization (cornification) of the vaginal mucosa.
- Enlargement of labia minora and majora.
- Uterine enlargement.
- Increased fat deposition in hips and thighs.

Somatic growth

The pubertal growth spurt in girls typically begins 2 years before it begins in boys, accounting for about 50% of the 12 cm difference in average height between men and women. The other 50% results from a slower rate of growth during the spurt in girls compared with boys. The mechanisms by which sex steroids induce bone growth in girls are the same as in boys (Chapter 12). Structural growth ceases at a median age of 17 years in girls.

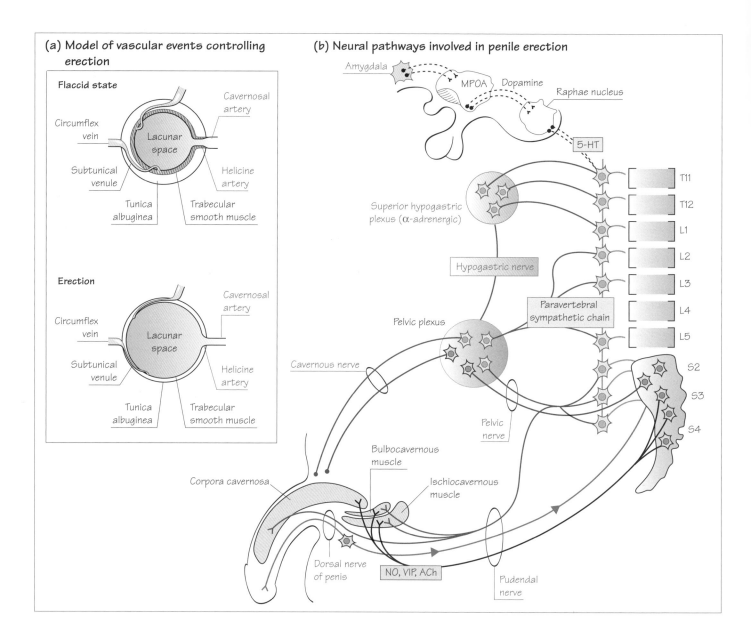

(a) Model of vascular events controlling erection

Flaccid state

- Circumflex vein
- Subtunical venule
- Tunica albuginea
- Lacunar space
- Cavernosal artery
- Helicine artery
- Trabecular smooth muscle

Erection

- Circumflex vein
- Subtunical venule
- Tunica albuginea
- Lacunar space
- Cavernosal artery
- Helicine artery
- Trabecular smooth muscle

(b) Neural pathways involved in penile erection

- Amygdala
- MPOA
- Dopamine
- Raphae nucleus
- 5-HT
- T11
- T12
- L1
- L2
- L3
- L4
- L5
- S2
- S3
- S4
- Superior hypogastric plexus (α-adrenergic)
- Hypogastric nerve
- Pelvic plexus
- Paravertebral sympathetic chain
- Cavernous nerve
- Pelvic nerve
- Corpora cavernosa
- Bulbocavernous muscle
- Ischiocavernous muscle
- Dorsal nerve of penis
- NO, VIP, ACh
- Pudendal nerve

Erection, emission and ejaculation

An **erection** is a complex neuropsychological event. It occurs when blood rapidly flows into the penis and becomes trapped in its spongy chambers. The three systems directly involved in a penile erection are (i) the spongy corpora cavernosa, (ii) the autonomic innervation of the penis and (iii) the blood supply of the penis. Sensory, peripheral and central nervous system pathways integrate the response.

Although there are three erectile bodies within the penis, the two corpora cavernosa are primarily responsible for penile rigidity during an erection. The corpus spongiosum becomes tumescent during an erection, but does not become rigid. It serves to redistribute the intraurethral pressure so that the urethra remains patent and an effective conduit for the ejaculate.

The basic physiology of an erection is best understood if one considers each corpus cavernosum as if it were a single lacunar chamber [see part (a) of figure]. Small (helicine) arteries transmit blood into the lacunar space, which is bounded by smooth muscle within the trabecular wall. These arteries have rigid, muscular walls. Exiting from the lacunar space are small venules that coalesce into larger (subtunical) venules. The subtunical venules drain through the tunica albuginea and form the emissary veins. Unlike arteries, veins have very flexible walls and are readily compressed.

When the penis is flaccid, the smooth muscle in the lacunar walls is in a contracted state. This contracted state is maintained by noradrenergic sympathetic fibres. Noradrenergic tone is blocked upon activation of the parasympathetic system and the intralacunar smooth muscle relaxes.

Blood flows easily into the relaxed lacunar space through the helicine arteries. This distends the lacunar space and the subtunical venules and emissary veins are physically compressed by the expanded lacunae. In essence, the lacunar space becomes a large vascular 'sink'. Blood readily flows into this sink, but it is unable to exit via the penile venous system. Distension increases until the intralacunar pressure equals the mean arterial pressure.

Regulation of cavernosal smooth muscle is central to control of an erection. Simultaneous parasympathetic neural pathway activation and inhibition of sympathetic outflow are required for the smooth muscle relaxation that allows blood to flow into the sinusoidal spaces. The parasympathetic nervous innervation travels to the penis through the pelvic nerve whereas the sympathetic innervation travels in the hypogastric nerve. Numerous neurotransmitters are involved in the parasympathetic modulation of cavernosal smooth muscle relaxation. **Nitric oxide is the primary pro-erectile neurotransmitter**. It colocalizes with acetylcholine and vasoactive intestinal peptide (VIP) in nerve fibres terminating on the trabeculae of the corpora cavernosa and on the helicine arteries. Cavernosal smooth muscle contraction appears to be largely under α-noradrenergic control. Norepinephrine is the major anti-erectile agent.

Reflex erection can be elicited by afferent signals from sensory nerve endings on the glans; this reflex is mediated at the level of the spinal cord. The afferent limb of the reflex is carried by the internal pudendal nerves, which can also be activated by tactile stimulation of the perineum near the testes and scrotum. Erections can be modulated by supraspinal influences in the central nervous system. For instance, serotonergic pathways within the raphe nucleus of the midbrain can inhibit erections. The amygdala and the medial preoptic area of the hypothalamus appear to be important higher integrating centres. Dopamine is the candidate neurotransmitter in erectile control at this level.

The importance of testosterone in erectile function is not known. Nocturnal erections, which occur during episodes of rapid eye movement (REM) sleep, are testosterone dependent. In contrast, erections that occur in response to visual stimuli are not dependent on testosterone and will occur in hypogonadal men.

As ejaculation approaches, penile turgor increases even more. The smooth muscles in the prostate, vas deferens and seminal vesicles contract sequentially to expel the seminal plasma and spermatozoa into the urethra in a process known as **emission**. Emission is mediated by α-adrenergic sympathetic fibres that travel through the hypogastric nerve. Ejaculation is distinct from emission and is characterized by the ejection of semen from the posterior urethra. **Ejaculation** requires contraction of the smooth muscles of the urethra and the striated bulbocavernosis and ischiocavernosis muscles.

Hormonal control of spermatogenesis

Although ongoing spermatogenesis in the testes can be maintained qualitatively by testosterone alone, follicle-stimulating hormone (FSH) is required for initiation of spermatogenesis. The primary site of action of FSH within the seminiferous epithelium is in the Sertoli cells.

FSH is delivered to the interstitial area of the testis via small arterioles. Once there, it diffuses through the basement membrane of the seminiferous tubules and binds to specific plasma membrane receptors on Sertoli cells. Activation of the FSH receptors results in the synthesis of both intracellular androgen receptors and androgen-binding protein (ABP). ABP is secreted from the Sertoli cells and binds androgens that have been produced by Leydig cells and diffused from their interstitial site of production into the seminiferous tubule. ABP transfers these androgens to the germ cells. Here, the androgens will be retained in the promeiotic germ cells that contain androgen receptors. Once FSH initiates spermatogenesis, the process will proceed as long as an adequate and uninterrupted supply of testosterone is available.

The FSH dependence of the Sertoli cells is analogous to the FSH control of the homologous granulosa cells in the ovary. Like follicular phase ovarian granulosa cells, Sertoli cells also secrete inhibin and activin. Inhibin, along with testosterone, inhibits pituitary FSH secretion in the male. Activin receptors have been identified on spermatogenic cells and may be involved in the FSH-mediated initiation of spermatogenesis.

Leydig cell function

Like the homologous theca cells in the ovary, Leydig cells respond to LH by synthesizing and secreting testosterone in a dose-dependent manner. In addition to LH receptors, receptors for prolactin and inhibin are found on Leydig cells. Both prolactin and inhibin facilitate the stimulatory activity of LH on testosterone production; neither can do this in isolation.

Regulation of gonadotropin secretion in males

The neuroendocrine mechanisms that regulate testicular function are fundamentally similar to those that regulate ovarian function. Hypothalamic GnRH, secreted in a pulsatile fashion into the pituitary portal system, acts on the pituitary of the male to stimulate synthesis and release of the gonadotropins, FSH and LH. These two gonadotropins regulate the spermatogenic and endocrine activities of the testis. The male and female utilize the same negative feedback mechanisms to inhibit gonadotropin release by the pituitary. There is, however, a major difference between regulation of the male and female hypothalamic–pituitary–gonadal systems. The postpubertal male has continuous gametogenesis and testosterone production while the postpubertal female has cyclic functions. The lack of cyclicity in males occurs because androgens do not exert a positive feedback on gonadotropin release.

Testosterone is the major regulator of LH secretion in the male. The negative feedback effect of testosterone is achieved largely by decreasing the frequency of the GnRH pulses released by the hypothalamus; although there are minor reductions in GnRH pulse amplitude. Testosterone also inhibits FSH release but its effects are not as pronounced as they are on LH. Combinations of testosterone and the Sertoli cell hormone inhibin (Chapter 2) are required to produce maximal FSH suppression.

The menstrual cycle

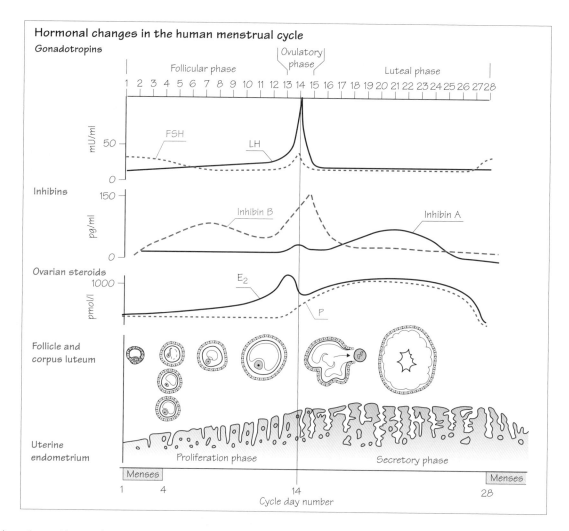

Hormonal changes in the human menstrual cycle

Gametogenesis and steroidogenesis proceed in a continuous fashion in the postpubertal human male. In contrast, the postpubertal human female exhibits repetitive cyclic changes in the hypothalamic–pituitary –ovarian axis that allow: (i) the maturation and release of gametes from the ovary and (ii) the development of a uterine environment prepared to support a pregnancy should fertilization occur. In the absence of conception, each cycle ends in menstrual bleeding. The pituitary gonadotropins, luteinizing hormone (LH) and follicle-stimulating hormone (FSH), link the hypothalamus and the ovary and mediate these cyclic changes.

The human menstrual cycle is best understood if divided into four phases based on functional and morphological changes in the ovary and endometrium: (i) follicular, (ii) ovulatory, (iii) luteal and (iv) menstrual.

Follicular phase

Conventionally considered the first phase, this is the phase of the menstrual cycle leading up to ovulation. In a typical 28-day menstrual cycle, it comprises the first 14 days. In ovulatory cycles of more or less than 28 days' duration, the deviation from the average is largely due to differences in the length of the follicular phase.

During this phase of the human menstrual cycle, a cohort of ovarian follicles will begin to mature, although only one typically

becomes the dominant follicle, called the **Graffian follicle**. Progression of follicles from their primordial or resting state in the ovary begins during the few days prior to initiation of menstruation in the previous cycle, although selection of which follicles will mature in a given cycle may occur several months prior to morphological recruitment. As one cycle ends, the programmed demise of the corpus luteum results in a rapid decline in its hormonal secretion. The resultant fall in serum oestradiol releases the central negative feedback inhibition on FSH secretion. Associated declines in progesterone and inhibin A are involved to a lesser degree. Increases in FSH secretion during the late luteal phase are accompanied by an increase in the pulse frequency of LH secretion.

Day 1 of menstrual bleeding is considered the first day of the follicular phase. During the first 4–5 days of the phase, development of the early ovarian follicle cohort is characterized by FSH-induced granulosa cell proliferation and aromatase activity. The theca cells of the developing follicle produce androgen precursors. These are converted into oestradiol within neighbouring granulosa cells. The process has been called the two-cell hypothesis. Oestradiol levels increase. The recruited follicles now have several layers of granulosa cells surrounding their oocytes and a small accumulation of follicular fluid. FSH induces synthesis of additional FSH receptors on granulosa cells, expanding its own effects. FSH also stimulates synthesis of new LH receptors on the granulosa cells, thereby initiating LH responsiveness.

By days 5–7 of the menstrual cycle, a single follicle predominates to the detriment of the others in the selected cohort, and will mature and ovulate between days 13 and 15. The predominant follicle is characterized by the highest mitotic index of all the recruited follicles, an optimal capacity for FSH retention in its follicular fluid, and high oestradiol and inhibin B synthesis. Non-dominant follicles have elevated androgen:oestrogen ratios in their follicular fluid, suggesting suboptimal induction of aromatase activity, and will undergo **atresia**. Androgens appear to be key to the atresia process, as granulosa cells treated with androgen *in vitro* undergo apoptosis.

During the mid- to late follicular phase, continued elevations in circulating oestradiol and inhibin B suppress FSH secretion, so preventing new follicular recruitment. Continuous high elevations of circulating oestradiol exert a somewhat unexpected effect on the pituitary gland: exponential increases in LH secretion. The ovary also exhibits increased responsiveness to the gonadotropins. Lastly, high oestrogen levels cause growth of the endometrial tissue lining the uterus. These changes in the endometrium can be distinguished microscopically and are defined as the 'proliferative phase' (Chapter 11).

Ovulatory phase

This phase of the menstrual cycle is characterized by a surge in pituitary LH secretion, culminating in extrusion of the mature ovum through the capsule of the ovary. In the 2–3 days preceding the onset of the LH surge, circulating oestradiol and inhibin B rise rapidly and in parallel. Oestradiol synthesis is at a maximum and no longer dependent on FSH. Progesterone begins to rise as the surging LH induces progesterone synthesis by the granulosa cells.

Key to ovulation is the midcycle positive feedback effect of oestrogen on LH secretion. Proof that rising ovarian oestrogens are central to ovulation lies in the observation that a gonadotropin surge can be elicited when prolonged elevated circulating oestradiol concentrations are produced experimentally by 2–3 days of exogenous oestrogen administration in women. The effects of elevated circulating oestrogen are further augmented by the presence of ovarian progesterone. The site of the positive feedback actions of midcycle oestrogen on LH secretion appears to be in both the hypothalamic neuroendocrine cells and the pituitary gonadotropes. The exact mechanism by which oestrogen induces the midcycle LH surge is uncertain, but dopaminergic and β-endorphinergic neuronal modulation of the GnRH pulse generator are involved. In fact, at midcycle, there is a 20-fold increase in sensitivity of the pituitary gonadotropes to GnRH. Further, the GnRH pulse generator can be inhibited by both synthetic and naturally occurring opioids, suggesting that opioids play a pivotal role in the neuronal control of the midcycle LH surge. A small rise in FSH occurs simultaneously with the pronounced rise in LH at midcycle, presumably in response to the GnRH signal.

Ovulation appears to require LH. The exact mechanism of this effect is unknown, although prostaglandins are thought to be at least one of the mediators. To this point, LH has been shown to stimulate prostaglandin biosynthesis by ovarian cells and inhibitors of prostaglandin synthesis inhibit ovulation in animals. Plasminogen activator may also be involved. Plasminogen activator, a serine protease that converts plasminogen to the proteolytically active enzyme plasmin, is produced by ovarian cells in response to FSH and may mediate the effects of the midcycle FSH surge on ovulation.

Luteal phase

After ovulation, the dominant morphological and functional feature of the ovary is the formation and maintenance of the corpus luteum. In humans, the luteal cells make large amounts of oestrogen and inhibin. In fact, the circulating oestrogen concentrations during the luteal phase are in the preovulatory, positive feedback range. Characteristic of the luteal phase, however, are the uniquely high concentrations of progesterone and 17-hydroxyprogesterone secreted by the corpus luteum. Progesterone at these elevated levels prevents oestrogen from stimulating another LH surge from the pituitary. Instead, in the presence of the combination of high concentrations of progesterone and oestrogen, the preovulatory GnRH pulses are reduced in frequency, resulting in only baseline FSH and LH secretion.

The length of the luteal phase is more consistent than that of the follicular phase, normally 14 ± 2 days. If pregnancy does not ensue, the corpus luteum spontaneously regresses and follicular development proceeds for the next cycle. Only small amounts of LH are necessary to maintain the corpus luteum in a normal cycle. However, after 14 days, even basal LH secretion will no longer support the endocrine function of the gland. If pregnancy ensues, maintenance of the corpus luteum and its progesterone production is critical to the success of the early gestation. Chorionic gonadotropin (hCG) is a hormone homologous to LH. hCG is secreted by the placental tissues (trophoblast) of a developing pregnancy. Therefore, in the presence of pregnancy, hCG secreted by gestational trophoblast can maintain the corpus luteum until the trophoblast assumes the role of progesterone secretion (Chapter 18). High levels of progesterone also create the 'secretory phase' of the endometrium, which is marked by endometrial maturation that can allow implantation of the embryo (Chapter 17). The exact trigger for the demise of the corpus luteum in a cycle that does not result in pregnancy is unknown. DNA fragmentation patterns characteristic of apoptosis appear in the corpus luteum as early as the mid- to late luteal phase.

The rise in FSH secretion near the end of the luteal phase is dependent on a concomitant drop in the high circulating levels of progesterone, oestradiol and inhibin. It is clinically significant that an oestrogen antagonist such as clomiphene citrate, administered in the luteal phase, causes a rise in circulating FSH levels and initiation of follicular recruitment.

Menstrual phase

The first day of menstruation marks the beginning of the next cycle. A new wave of follicles has been recruited and will progress toward maturation and, for one, ovulation. The phenomenon known as menstruation is largely an endometrial event, triggered by the loss of progesterone support from the corpus luteum in non-conception cycles.

Dramatic structural changes occur in the endometrium during menstruation, driven by complex and only partially understood mechanisms. Hormonally regulated matrix-degrading proteases and lysosomes appear to be involved. Matrix-degrading proteases are part of the metalloproteinase (MMP) family of enzymes whose substrates include collagen and other matrix proteins. Of the MMP family, seven members are expressed in cell- and menstrual cycle-specific patterns. Also, the endothelins, which are potent vasoconstrictors, appear to have maximum activity at the end of the luteal phase. Finally, the premenstrual fall in progesterone is associated with a decline in 15-hydroxyprostaglandin dehydrogenase activity. This results in an increase in the availability of prostaglandin $PGF_{2\alpha}$, a potent stimulator of myometrial contractility. Prostaglandin and thromboxane homeostasis direct myometrial and vascular contractions within the uterus. Control of such contractility is central to the creation of endometrial ischaemia, the promotion of endometrial sloughing and the cessation of menstrual bleeding.

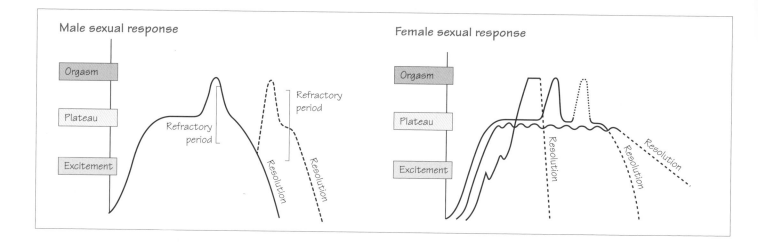

Successful reproduction is the ultimate definition of evolutionary fitness. Because fertilization occurs within the reproductive tract of humans, intimate contact between male and female is necessary for spontaneous conception to occur. Therefore, from an evolutionary view, human sexual behaviour should ultimately be directed toward the physiology of coitus, which results in the deposition of sperm within the female reproductive tract. Of course, this purely procreational approach to sexual behaviour is too simplistic. Humans differ from most animals, whose mating is seasonable and determined by hormonal cycles, in being sexually receptive regardless of fertility potential. Human sexuality is defined not only by procreation, but also by recreation and pleasure. The non-reproductive aspect of human sexuality is quite plastic and subject to individual and cultural influences. What is pleasurable to one individual may not be so to another. Normative behaviour in one culture may be unacceptable in another. What does seem to be common to all human sexual responses is that both physiological and psychological satisfaction are central and motivating.

Most sexual encounters pass through five stages. The first stage, sexual attraction or arousal, was not included in initial descriptions of the human sexual response cycle. The latter four stages were first defined by the pioneering work of Masters and Johnson. Using hundreds of observations made during heterosexual interactions and masturbation, they divided the human sexual response into excitement, plateau, orgasm and resolution phases. Although the validity of some of the data gathered by Masters and Johnson has been subject to question, their model remains the single best description of the physiological aspects of the human sexual response.

Phases of the sexual response

Sexual attraction or arousal is the most individualized stage of the human sexual response. In many respects, sexual attraction and arousal are closely tied to personality. They are also the most culturally determined. For example, incest taboos forbidding marriage and intercourse between closely related family members are almost universal among cultures over time. In contrast, attention to women's breasts or weight in a sexual context varies tremendously among cultures. Interestingly,

two variables of attractiveness do appear to be both universal and related to reproductive success: youth and health.

The nature of erotic stimuli can also be quite varied and include mental images, smells, sounds and physical events such as touching or stroking. If self-report and measurements of pelvic blood flow are used to indicate the level of arousal, men and women seem to be equally arousable. They differ dramatically, however, in the types of things that result in arousal. Novel or unpredictable situations and explicit visual stimuli, particularly body images, appeal to men more than women. Women generally prefer images with an emotional, romantic or familiar context. An individual's physical health and mental state contribute greatly to the threshold at which they can be aroused by a given stimulus.

During the next phase of the sexual response cycle, the physiological **excitement phase**, sexual interest is stimulated by these psychological or physiological stimuli. This aroused state intensifies during the **plateau phase**. If stimulation is sufficient, **orgasm** or climax occurs. Orgasm is typically experienced as an explosive and pleasant release of sexual tension. Finally, during the **resolution phase**, sexual arousal dissipates. The physiological changes associated with arousal and orgasm return to baseline. Although both men and women progress through the same phases of sexual response, they may differ in length and intensity in any given sexual encounter. The most notable physiological difference between males and females is the presence of a refractory period in men. This is a part of the resolution phase following orgasm. During this period of time, sexual arousal cannot be restored and orgasm cannot occur in men. In contrast, sufficient stimulation can induce orgasm in women at any point during the resolution phase.

The basic physiological responses of the human body to sexual stimulation are twofold. The primary reaction is **vascular congestion**. The secondary response is **generalized muscle tension** or myotonia. Reflexes activated within the spinal cord are modulated by the higher central nervous system and control each response.

Male sexual response

The human male's first physiological response to effective sexual stimulation is penile erection. Erection occurs during the excitement phase, with vasodilatation of the lacunar smooth muscle of the penis leading to its engorgement and hardening (Chapter 14). Only a minimal degree of sexual tension may accompany excitation and this phase of the sexual response can vary significantly in length.

Erectile stimuli may be either psychogenic or somatogenic. Psychogenic stimuli can include imagined sensory cues or direct visual cues, including explicitly erotic images. These signals are integrated within the limbic system of the brain and transmitted via descending projections to the spinal cord. They then travel via autonomic and visceral efferent nerves to the penis. Somatogenic stimuli include touching the penis or adjacent perineum. These tactile stimuli will reflexly activate the same efferents as the spinal cord pathway. This tactile reflex is typically preserved following spinal cord transection. The erection of the excitement phase may be quite susceptible to external signals and may resolve without progression. Changes in the physical surroundings, such as sudden loud noises, can impair penile erection in the excitation phase. Erection of the penis can also occur independent of the excitation phase of sexual arousal, observable in the newborn period and during sleep, especially in pubescent boys.

During the plateau phase, a minor involuntary increase in vasocongestion occurs and penile erection increases slightly. The size of the testes likewise increases and the scrotum and testes are drawn toward the perineum. There is a measurable rise in heart rate and systolic blood pressure. Just prior to ejaculation, a warm red rash may develop over the upper abdomen, trunk, neck and face. There is a diffuse and near-maximal increase in muscular tension throughout the body. Emission immediately precedes ejaculation. During emission, muscular contractions are induced within the prostate gland, vas deferens and seminal vesicles and seminal plasma and spermatozoa are expelled into the posterior urethra. This process is mediated by sympathetic output travelling through the hypogastric plexus and can be abolished by α-adrenergic blockade. Once the plateau phase is reached, detumescence without ejaculation and orgasm is rare in healthy individuals.

During orgasm, somatic changes in the cardiovascular system are at their maximum, as is generalized muscle tension. Hyperventilation and vocalizations are common. Contraction of the smooth muscles of the urethra and the striated muscles of the bulbocavernosus and ischiocavernosus muscles expels the semen from the prostatic urethra. The pelvic floor and rectal sphincter may contract rhythmically. **Ejaculation** of the semen from the penis marks the height of orgasm. It is typically accompanied by release of sexual tension and an intense sense of pleasure.

Penile detumescence during the **resolution phase** of the male sexual response cycle occurs in two distinct stages. The primary stage of penile involution occurs very rapidly. The penis reduces in size from full erection to about 50% larger than its flaccid, unstimulated size. The penis is totally refractory to stimulation during this first stage. Secondary stage involution is a more extended process that returns the penis to its normal unstimulated size. The penis is only relatively refractory to stimulation during this stage. The penis progressively regains responsiveness. The excitement or plateau phase of the sexual cycle may be voluntarily extended by the male in an effort to delay ejaculation until his sexual partner is satisfied. This may be accompanied by a prolongation of the primary stage of detumescence after ejaculation.

Female sexual response

During the excitement phase of the sexual response cycle, somatogenic and psychogenic stimuli arouse the female through neural pathways similar to those described for the male. The clitoral response to arousal is less predictable than is that of its homologue, the penis. Tactile stimulation of the female perineum or the glans clitoris can elicit vasocongestion, engorgement of the body of the clitoris and erection, but only in some women. The response of the vagina during the excitement phase is much more predictable and consistent than that of the clitoris. Vaginal lubrication begins 10–30 s after receipt of arousing stimuli and continues progressively through orgasm. The more prolonged the excitement and plateau phases, the greater the production of vaginal lubrication. The upper two-thirds of the vagina also expand and lengthen during the excitement phase. This elevates the uterus into the false pelvis, repositions the cervix above the vaginal floor and 'tents' the midvaginal plane. These changes result in an increase in the circumference of the vaginal diameter, largely at the level of the cervix. Finally, the labia minora become markedly engorged with blood during the excitement phase. The engorged labia minora displace the labia majora upward and outward away from the vaginal introitus. This increase in the diameter of the labia minora adds at least 1 cm to the functional length of the vagina.

During the plateau phase, the most striking change in the female genitalia is the florid coloration of the labia minora accompanying vascular congestion. This beet red appearance is the single most consistent physical marker for sexual arousal in the female. The clitoris retracts behind a tissue hood formed by the labia. The respiratory rate, heart rate and blood pressure all increase late in the plateau phase; the magnitude of these changes are not as marked in women as in men. Generalized myotonia may be present, including spastic contractions of the striated muscles of the hands and feet. The latter are referred to as carpopedal spasms.

During heterosexual coitus, penetration of the penis into the vagina can heighten a woman's sexual arousal by indirectly stimulating the retracted clitoris. This occurs because of traction on the engorged labia minora whose fused anterior segment forms the clitoral hood. The glans of the clitoris, however, is extremely sensitive in the aroused state. For this reason, direct and prolonged contact may be irritating.

Similar to the male, orgasm in the female involves rhythmic contractions of the muscles of the reproductive organs followed by physical release from the vasocongestive and myotonic tensions developed during arousal. Typically, orgasmic contractions begin in the lower third of the vagina and evolve to encompass the entire vagina and uterus. A sex flush, which can also include diffuse fine perspiration, may develop over the woman's entire body. The resolution phase of the sexual response cycle of women involves decongestion of the labia, detumescence of the clitoris if it has occurred, and relaxation of the vagina.

There are three major physiological differences between male and female orgasms. First, emission and ejaculation do not occur in the female. Second, if sexual stimulation occurs before a woman drops below plateau phase levels of arousal, the female is capable of rapidly successive orgasms. Finally, the female orgasm may last for a relatively long period compared to that of the male.

17 Fertilization and the establishment of pregnancy

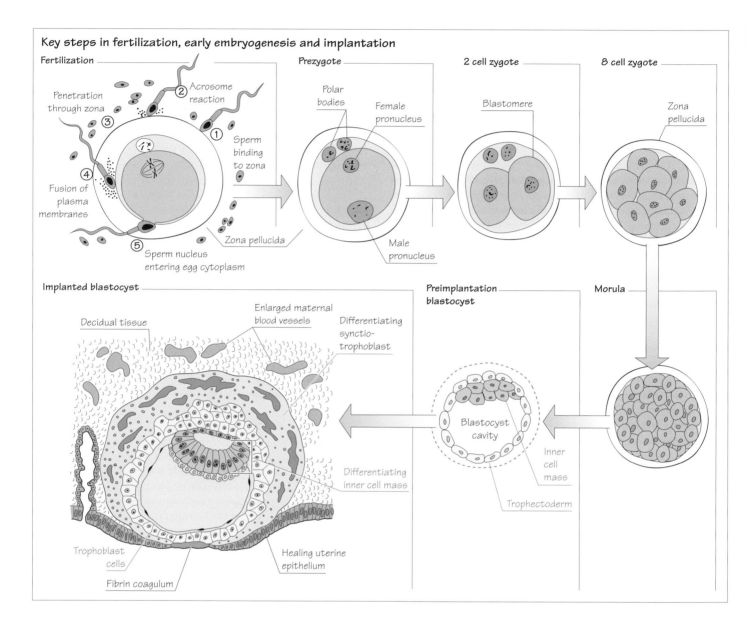

The egg

At ovulation, the egg is arrested in metaphase of the second meiotic division. It is surrounded by a proteinaceous sphere called the **zona pellucida**. Those granulosa cells that adhered to the surface of the zona pellucida and were expelled with the egg from the ovary remain attached as the cumulus. Sperm that ultimately fertilize the egg must first negotiate these surrounding layers before they can penetrate the egg cell membrane. The oocyte will remain viable for 6–24 h once ovulated.

The sperm

With coitus, millions of sperm are deposited in the upper vagina. Most will never arrive at the site of fertilization. Abnormal sperm can rarely make this long trip successfully and even most of the healthy spermatozoa die along the way. The vast majority leak from the vagina upon liquification of the semen. Only a small proportion enter the cervix,

where they will be found within minutes of coitus. Here they can survive within the epithelial crypts for hours. Sperm cannot traverse the cervix into the uterine cavity unless the cervical mucous is receptive. This typically occurs at midcycle when oestrogen levels are high and progesterone is low. Oestrogen softens the cervical stroma and makes cervical secretions thin and watery. Progesterone has opposite effects, a combination hostile to spermatozoa.

In the best of conditions, it takes 2–7 h for sperm to move through the uterus to the site of fertilization within the oviduct. Sperm transport results from self-propulsion, aided by the ciliary beating of cells within the uterine lining. Typically only several hundred sperm reach the oviducts, where they will linger in a quiet state until ovulation occurs. After ovulation, these spermatozoa are reactivated and begin moving toward the egg. The signal that attracts the sperm to the egg is unknown. Human spermatozoa can survive for a total of 24–48 h in the female reproductive tract.

Freshly ejaculated spermatozoa are not capable of fertilizing an egg. They acquire the ability to penetrate the cell layers surrounding the oocyte through a process known as **capacitation**. Although capacitation can be induced *in vitro* under the proper culture conditions, it occurs *in vivo* within the female reproductive tract. During capacitation, the glycoprotein coat that adheres to the spermatozoa cell membranes is initially removed, initiating changes in the surface charge of the sperm membrane and reorganization of that membrane. Capacitated sperm change their tail movements from regular undulating waves to whip-like, thrashing movements that propel the sperm forward. At the biochemical level, capacitated sperm acquire increased calcium sensitivity and elevated internal cAMP levels. Capacitation takes several hours both *in vivo* and *in vitro*.

Sperm capacitation allows for the **acrosome reaction**. In the absence of an acrosome reaction, a sperm is incapable of penetrating the zona pellucida. Contact of an intact, capacitated sperm with the zona pellucida of an egg allows interaction of a specific sperm cell surface glycoprotein, ZP3, with specific zona protein. ZP3-binding induces further calcium influx into the spermatozoa and intracellular cAMP levels rise. The acrosome swells, its outer membrane fuses with the sperm plasma membrane, and the enzymatic contents of the acrosome are released into the extracellular space surrounding the head of the sperm. This also exposes the inner acrosomal membrane and another zona-binding protein, ZP2, to the oocyte zona. ZP2-binding holds sperm near the egg. Proteolytic enzymes released from the acrosome then facilitate penetration of the zona pellucida by the whiplashing sperm. Complete penetration of the zona takes about 15 min.

Fertilization

Penetration of the zona pellucida allows contact between spermatozoa and the oocyte membrane. The germ cell membranes fuse almost immediately and the sperm cell stops moving. The sperm nucleus enters the egg cytoplasm.

Three important events are triggered within the oocyte by the rise in intracellular calcium that occurs in the oocyte upon fusion of sperm and egg cell membranes. The egg cell membrane depolarizes, preventing membrane fusion with additional spermatozoa. This is the **primary block to polyspermy**. It assures that only one male pronucleus is available for fusion with the female pronucleus and protects the diploid status of the zygote. The second event is known as the **cortical reaction**. Cortical granules lie just beneath the egg cell membrane, and with the cortical reaction they fuse with the membrane and release their contents into the zona pellucida. This hardens the zona and impairs the ability of sperm to bind the zona—a **secondary block to polyspermy**. The third event involves resumption of the second meiotic division of the egg. The second polar body is formed and extruded from the egg, thereby assuring that the female pronucleus is haploid. Again, the diploid zygote is protected. Failure to preserve the diploid state of the conceptus is a frequent cause of early pregnancy failure (Chapter 36).

Upon entry into the egg, sperm cytoplasm mixes with that of the egg and the sperm nuclear membrane breaks down. A new membrane forms around the sperm chromatin, forming the **male pronucleus**. A new oocyte nuclear membrane also forms around the **female pronucleus**. DNA synthesis begins during this period as the haploid pronuclei prepare for the first mitotic division of the zygote. The pronuclear membranes break down, the parental chromosomes mix and the metaphase mitotic spindle forms. At about 24 h after fertilization, the chromosomes separate and the first cell division occurs.

During the first few embryonic cell divisions, no new mRNA is synthesized from the nuclear DNA of the conceptus. The embryo stays the same total size and the size of each individual cell decreases accordingly. Thus, the early embryo uses only maternal cell components to develop and important signals must be transmitted to the embryo through the oocyte cytoplasm. These signals likely reside in **mitochondrial DNA**, which *is* replicated during early embryonic cell division. In fact, mitochondrial DNA is quite stable and can be traced through generations to determine maternal lineage.

The establishment of pregnancy

After fertilization, a successful pregnancy must implant within the wall of the uterus and inform the mother that pregnancy adaptations must occur. Without these two important events, the zygote will simply wash out of the uterus with the next menses.

The cleaving zygote floats in the oviduct for approximately 1 week, progressing from the 16-cell stage through the solid **morula** (mulberry) stage to the 32–64-cell **blastocyst stage**. The latter stage requires formation of the fluid-containing blastocyst cavity. The blastocyst contains two distinct differentiated embryonic cell types: the outer **trophectoderm** cells and the **inner cell mass**. The trophectoderm cells will eventually form the placenta. The inner cell mass will form the fetus and fetal membranes. It is at the blastocyst stage that the conceptus enters the uterus.

During the time that it spends in the oviduct, the conceptus remains surrounded by the zona pellucida. After about 2 days in the uterus, the blastocyst will lose or 'hatch' from the zona pellucida. With hatching, the trophectodermal cells of the blastocyst begin to differentiate into **trophoblast** cells. These simultaneous processes allow trophoblast cells to make direct contact with the uterine luminal epithelial cells. The blastocyst attaches to and invades the uterine lining. Within hours, the surface epithelium immediately underlying the conceptus becomes eroded and nearby cells lyse, releasing primary metabolic substrates for use by the blastocyst. The endometrium undergoes dramatic biochemical and morphological changes called **decidualization**, a process that begins at the point of attachment and spreads out in a concentric wave from the point of implantation. The endometrium will heal over the conceptus so that the entire implantation becomes buried within the endometrium.

As the embryo invades maternal tissues the trophoblast cells further differentiate into two cell types: **cytotrophoblast cells** and **syncytiotrophoblast cells**. Syncytiotrophoblast cells are large, multinucleated cells that develop from the cytotrophoblast layer. They are active in placental hormone secretion and in nutrient transport from mother to fetus. A subset of cytotrophoblast cells acquire invasive properties, traversing endometrial stroma to reach maternal blood vessels, including the spiral arteries of the endometrium. Appropriate invasion of the spiral arteries is key to a normal pregnancy outcome (Chapter 37).

A number of growth factors are integral to successful implantation. These include: (i) leukaemia inhibitory factor, a cytokine; (ii) the integrins, which mediate cell–cell interactions; and (iii) transforming growth factor beta (TGF-β), which stimulates syncytium formation and inhibits trophoblast invasion. Epidermal growth factor and interleukin 1β are important mediators of trophoblast invasion.

Implantation occurs about 7–10 days after ovulation. If the conceptus is to survive more than 14 days after ovulation, the ovarian corpus luteum must continue to secrete progesterone. **Human chorionic gonadotropin** (hCG) produced by the developing trophoblast and secreted into the maternal bloodstream acts like luteinizing hormone, supporting the corpus luteum by inhibiting luteal regression (Chapter 18).

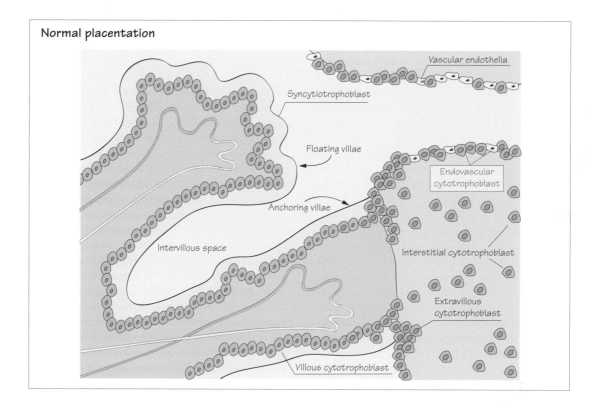

Normal placentation

Vascular endothelia

Syncytiotrophoblast

Floating villae

Endovascular cytotrophoblast

Anchoring villae

Interstitial cytotrophoblast

Intervillous space

Extravillous cytotrophoblast

Villous cytotrophoblast

Overview

The human placenta is the sole interface between the mother and her developing embryo/fetus. Humans differ from most other mammals in that maternal blood comes into direct contact with fetally derived placental tissues. This organization characterizes the haemochorial placenta through which all maternal nutrients and fetal wastes must pass. The placenta is a very active organ that has specialized mechanisms to promote fetal growth and survival. These include, but are not limited to, efficient gas exchange, active transport of energy substrates, immunological tolerance of the fetal allograft and fetal acquisition of maternal immunity.

Placental morphology

After it enters the uterus, the human blastocyst resides within the uterine cavity for 2–3 days prior to implantation into the decidualized uterine endometrium. Implantation can be divided into three distinct processes: apposition of the blastocyst to the endometrial epithelium at the site of implantation, a brief period of stable adhesion of the blastocyst to this epithelium, and invasion of the developing embryo into the uterine decidua. The signals governing these processes are complex and involve active maternal and fetal participation. **Apposition** requires the secretion of soluble mediators by uterine epithelia and the blastocyst that may include interleukins, prostaglandins and leukemia inhibiting factor (LIF). **Adhesion** is promoted by the expression of ligands on the surface of the developing embryo that specifically bind to receptors expressed on the uterine lining at the site of implantation. One receptor–ligand pair that has been implicated in embryo adhesion is heparin-binding epidermal growth factor and heparin sulfate proteoglycans. Also important in the adhesion process is a family of adhesion molecules

expressed on uterine epithelia in a time-specific and hormone-dependent fashion: the integrins. **Invasion** of the blastocyst into the maternal uterine decidua requires an alteration in the expression of embryonic surface molecules, from those promoting adhesion to the endometrium to others that stimulate invasion of vascular structures. During invasion, the embryo also begins to secrete proteases that digest between the cells of the decidua and allow invasion to areas deep within the uterine lining.

The developing embryo is comprised of two populations of cells (see figure in Chapter 17): one will become the fetus, the other, the placenta. At the blastocyst stage, the embryo is characterized by a fluid-filled cavity (the blastocoele), surrounded by a layer of trophectoderm cells. The trophectoderm will develop into the placenta. Within the trophectoderm shell is a collection of cells called the inner cell mass. All non-placental fetal tissues will arise from the inner cell mass.

During implantation, trophectoderm cells begin to differentiate into cellular subtypes that will characterize the mature placenta. The mature placenta is comprised of a mass of tree-like placental cotyledons called villae, which are bathed in maternal blood. Blood enters the space between the villae through low-resistance, high-flow vessels that branch from the maternal uterine spiral arteries. Fetal vessels are located within the core of each placental cotyledon. Loose connective tissue and layers of trophoblast cells surround each fetal vessel. The inner layers of the trophoblast shell around the vessels are called **cytotrophoblast** cells. The outer layer of the placental villae is coated by a multinucleated syncytium of fused trophoblast cells called the **syncytiotrophoblast**. The syncytiotrophoblast cells are directly bathed in maternal blood in the mature placenta.

The vast majority of placental cotyledons/villae float freely in the intervillous space. Here, they are surrounded by maternal blood. A

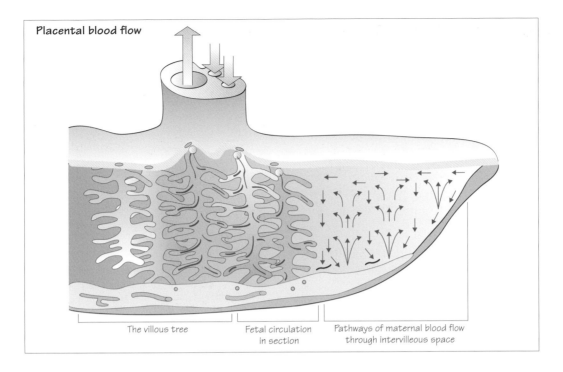

Placental blood flow

The villous tree | Fetal circulation in section | Pathways of maternal blood flow through intervilleous space

subset of villae completely cross the intervillous space and attach to the maternal uterine decidua. These are called anchoring villae. At the maternal end of the anchoring villae, a subset of cytotrophoblast cells change their phenotype and invade deep into the uterine lining. These extravillous cytotrophoblast cells come into direct contact with the maternal decidual immune cells that include a small number of B lymphocytes, a moderate number of T lymphocytes and macrophages, and a voluminous number of natural killer cells. A subset of extra-villous cytotrophoblast cells will invade directly into the maternal vasculature. These are the endovascular cytotrophoblast cells. They replace the endothelial cells of maternal vessels and transform the decidual vessels into the low-resistance, high-flow structures character-istic of a healthy, mature placenta.

Like the fetus, the placenta grows in size throughout pregnancy. At term, it is a large, beefy structure. Its maternal surface is covered with numerous cotyledons containing millions of villae. The fetal surface is covered with a smooth, glistening membrane called the amnion. The umbilical cord inserts almost perpendicularly into the fetal surface of the placenta.

Placental immunology

The maternal–fetal interface of the human haemochorial placenta allows direct exposure of fetally derived tissue to the maternal immune system. The fetal tissue, which contains both a maternal and paternal haplotype, is a hemi-allograft. Typically, when an immunocompetent organism encounters genetically foreign tissue, rejection occurs. This does not happen in pregnancy. Maternal immunological tolerance to the fetal allograft remains incompletely understood. Alterations in maternal immune responsivity may occur because of the maternal reproductive hormones. Progesterone and prolactin have remarkable immunosup-pressive activities and both are elevated in pregnancy. Also, the villous cytotrophoblast cells of the placenta do not express major histocom-patability complex (MHC) class I and MHC class II transplantation antigens on their surfaces. Extravillous cytotrophoblast cells also lack MHC class II antigens but express a unique subset of non-classical

MHC class I products. These non-classical products are thought to be important in interactions between placental cells and the very unique populations of immune cells residing at the site of implantation. Placental tissues may also have altered metabolic processes that promote immunosuppression. For instance, placental tissues rapidly degrade tryptophan, an amino acid that activates T lymphocytes.

Placental function

The placenta must supply the embryo and fetus with everything that it needs to grow and mature. Many complex systems exist within placental tissues to facilitate movement of nutrients into the fetus and wastes out. Driven by systemic blood pressure, maternal arterial blood spurts from the spiral arteries into the intervillous spaces and then disperses later-ally. The blood nearest the maternal decidua is under the least pressure and drains back into the maternal circulation. Only a fraction of the maternal blood vessels appear to spurt at any one time. This implies that that placental perfusion does not involve the entire placenta at any one time and that there is reserve capacity if a small separation from the uterine wall should occur.

At least four types of transport mechanisms move critical molecules from maternal blood, into the placenta and subsequently into the fetal circulation. Respiratory gas exchange occurs by concurrent passive diffusion down a concentration gradient as described by the Fick principle—its rate is proportional to the area of exchange, the dif-fusional permeability and the maternal and fetal blood flows. Although the oxygen content of umbilical cord blood coming directly from the placenta is low ($Po_2 = 28$–32 torr), the high affinity of fetal haemoglobin for oxygen assures that the fetal red blood cells are highly saturated with oxygen. Glucose, the primary metabolic fuel for the embryo and fetus, is transferred by facilitated diffusion involving classic GLUT transporters. Calcium enters the placenta through active cation transport whereas many amino acids are transported against concentration gradients coupled to sodium transport. Immunoglobulins of the IgG class enter the placenta through endocytosis following binding of the Fc end of the Ig G molecules to membrane Fc receptors on trophoblasts.

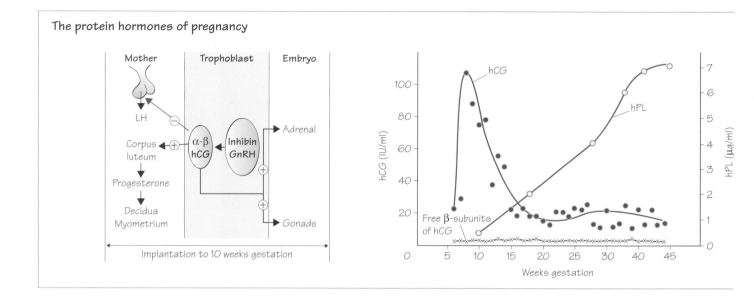

The protein hormones of pregnancy

Placental production of protein hormones

The placenta is a very rich source of both protein and steroid hormones, only a few of which are unique to pregnancy. These placental hormones are responsible for almost all the maternal and some of the fetal adaptations to pregnancy.

Human chorionic gonadotropin

Human chorionic gonadotropin (hCG) is a dimeric protein hormone whose structure is closely related to luteinizing hormone (LH) (Chapter 2). It is among the earliest products of the trophoblast cells of the embryo and is necessary to signal the maternal organism that conception has occurred. β-hCG mRNA can be detected in an eight-cell embryo, although intact hCG is not detectable in the maternal bloodstream or urine until 6 days after fertilization. hCG secretion is quantitatively related to the total mass of cytotrophoblast cells in the placenta. Its concentration in the maternal serum doubles every 2–3 days in early pregnancy; this can be used as a screen to differentiate normal from abnormal pregnancies. Failure of the hCG concentrations to increase appropriately may indicate an abnormal implantation such as an ectopic (tubal) pregnancy or a non-viable intrauterine gestation. Higher than expected levels of hCG are seen with multiple gestations and molar pregnancies.

The major biological role of hCG is to 'rescue' the corpus luteum of the ovary from its programmed demise 12–14 days after ovulation. Because of the close structural relationship of hCG to LH, hCG is able to bind to the LH receptor on luteal cells. hCG can therefore substitute for LH, supporting the corpus luteum when a pregnancy is present. Maintenance of the corpus luteum allows continued secretion of ovarian progesterone after day 14 post-ovulation and maintenance of the early pregnancy. Surgical removal of the corpus luteum without progesterone supplementation or before the 9th menstrual week of pregnancy will result in a pregnancy loss. Administration of an antiprogestin such as

RU-486 will have similar results. By 9 weeks of gestation (7 weeks after conception), the placenta has acquired sufficient cellular mass to supply the large amounts of progesterone necessary for pregnancy maintenance. Progesterone production is taken over by the placenta and the corpus luteum could be removed without adverse effect on pregnancy maintenance. At the end of the first trimester, hCG also stimulates the fetal gonads to make the steroid hormones responsible for differentiation of the internal and external genitalia (Chapters 6 and 7).

Many of the hormones produced within the placenta result from a two-cell system that mimics the interactions between the neuroendocrine hypothalamus and the pituitary gland. For instance, gonadotropin-releasing hormone (GnRH) can be synthesized and secreted by the cytotrophoblast cells of the placenta. GnRH from the cytotrophoblast stimulates hCG production by the syncytiotrophoblast. As pregnancy progresses and the placenta becomes the major site of progesterone production, hCG's primary role changes from maintenance of the corpus luteum to maintenance of progesterone production by the syncytiotrophoblast. The serum level of hCG reflects this change by increasing to a maximum at about the 7th menstrual week of pregnancy and then decreasing to a much lower steady state level for the remainder of the pregnancy.

Human placental lactogen

Human placental lactogen (hPL) is a protein hormone produced exclusively by the placenta. It is structurally related to both prolactin and growth hormone (GH). When the peptide was originally isolated from the placenta, its biological activity was assessed in animal models where it has lactogenic activity. Although it was designated as a lactogen, lactogenic activity has not been clearly demonstrated in the human. Instead, hPL appears to function in metabolism. Its metabolic activities closely mimic those of GH, with which it shares 96% structural homology. Its effects on fat and carbohydrate metabolism include inhibition of peripheral glucose uptake, stimulation of insulin

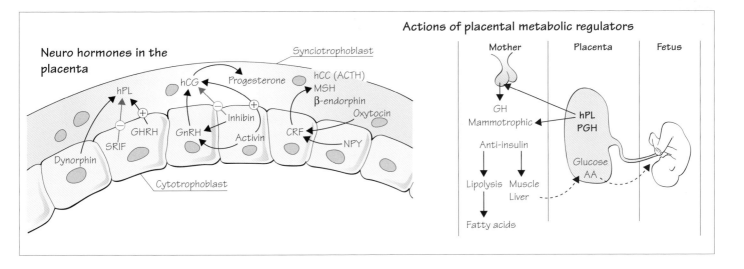

release by the pancreas and an increase in plasma free fatty acids. Prolonged fasting and hypoglycaemia increase hPL production. During pregnancy, blood glucose decreases, insulin secretion increases, and peripheral insulin resistance is enhanced. These metabolic changes are consistent with the presence of increased GH-like activity, possibly the effects of hPL. Another name for hPL is **human chorionic somatomammotropin (hCS)**.

In theory, the decreased maternal glucose utilization induced by hPL would ensure that a steady supply of glucose is available for fetal utilization. There is growing evidence that hPL is involved in regulating glucose homeostasis in the mother so that she can meet the nutritional demands of the fetus; although successful pregnancies have been reported in the absence of hPL production by the placenta. In normal pregnancies, hPL production is directly proportional to placental mass and, therefore, rises steadily throughout pregnancy. At the end of gestation, over 1 g per day of hPL is produced by the placenta. This amount surpasses the production levels of any other protein hormone in either men or women.

Other hormones

Pituitary growth hormone of either maternal or fetal origin is not necessary for normal fetal growth. In fact, anencephalic fetuses lacking a pituitary gland and the offspring of women with growth hormone deficiency will grow normally *in utero*. The placenta produces its own variant of growth hormone protein, known as **placental growth hormone (PGH)**. PGH is a candidate hormone for regulating fetal growth.

Both the cytotrophoblast and syncytiotrophoblast cells secrete **corticotropin-releasing hormone (CRH)** and **pro-opiomelanocortin (POM-C)**, the precursor of **adrenocorticotropic hormone (ACTH)**. Maternal CRH levels and placental CRH content rise in the last month

of pregnancy. Glucocorticoids enhance CRH mRNA production by the placenta, suggesting a positive feedback system. It is hypothesized that placental CRH and ACTH may be involved in the timing of the onset of parturition.

Maternal production of protein hormones

Placental hormones exert dramatic effects on the production and activities of non-placental maternal protein hormones. For example, placental oestrogen production stimulates the production of many hepatic proteins. Among these is thyroid-binding globulin (TBG). The increase in circulating TBG in the pregnant woman leaves less thyroid hormone free to circulate. Because free thyroid hormone exerts central negative feedback, this decrease in free thyroid hormone frees the hypothalamus to release thyroid-releasing hormone (TRH). Maternal pituitary thyroid-stimulating hormone (TSH) secretion increases in response to TRH and the maternal thyroid gland produces enough T_3 and T_4 to return the circulating levels to normal. Pregnant women therefore have higher levels of TBG, total T_3 and T_4, but normal amounts of free T_3 and T_4. This can cause confusion when interpreting thyroid function tests in pregnancy. It also means that pregnant women taking hormone replacement for thyroid gland deficiency often need to increase their dose to maintain adequate free hormone levels.

Pituitary production of prolactin also increases dramatically as a result of oestrogen stimulation in the pregnant woman. The number of lactotrophs in the pituitary gland doubles, thereby almost doubling the size and blood supply of the pituitary gland. This increase in size makes the pituitary gland particularly vulnerable to ischaemic damage. Therefore, if postpartum haemorrhage and shock are not promptly treated, pituitary gland failure (Sheehan syndrome) may develop.

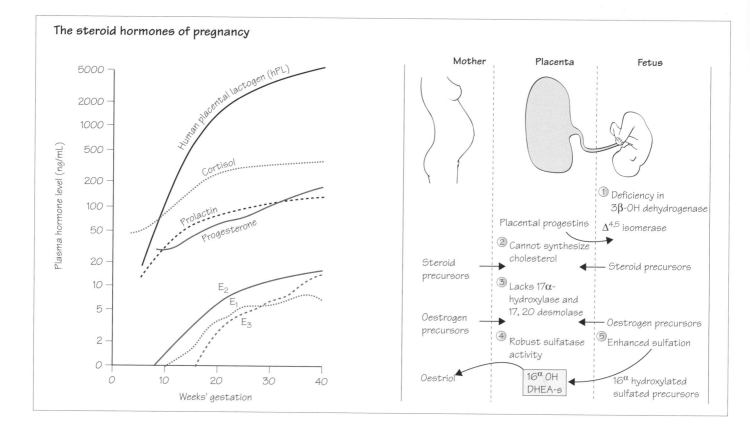

The steroid hormones of pregnancy

Steroid hormone production during pregnancy requires cooperation among maternal, fetal and placental organs and enzyme pathways. The fetus and the placenta each lack key steroidogenic enzymes and would be unable to synthesize certain steroid molecules if they existed in isolation. Interplay among fetus, placenta and the mother are essential to produce the full spectrum of steroidal products necessary for pregnancy maintenance. For example, the fetal adrenal gland has diminished 3β-hydroxysteroid dehydrogenase: Δ^{4-5} isomerase activity and therefore it secretes large amounts of the progesterone precursors, pregnenolone and dehydroepiandrosterone, and very little progesterone (Chapter 3). Because the fetus can synthesize so very little progesterone directly, it obtains its supplies from the placenta. Because the syncytiotrophoblast cells of the placenta lack a key enzyme, they cannot synthesize cholesterol from circulating acetate. To synthesize progesterone, the placenta requires cholesterol or pregnenolone from maternal or fetal sources. The vast majority arises from the maternal system and is transported to the placenta in the form of low density lipoprotein (LDL)-cholesterol. In contrast to the mother and placenta, the fetus has a remarkable ability to rapidly conjugate steroids with sulfates. Sulfation creates less potent steroids with more rapid clearance, characteristics that allow the fetus to be safely exposed to the high levels of circulating steroids seen during pregnancy. The fetal liver can efficiently hydroxylate steroid precursors and thereby provides the placenta with those hydroxylated steroids necessary for oestrogen production. The placenta has almost no 17α-hydroxylase or 17–20 desmolase activity. For this reason, the precursors of the oestrogens produced by the placenta must be supplied by the fetal or maternal

systems. The placenta exhibits a robust ability to cleave sulfate groups from steroids. Placental sulfatase is integral to the formation of oestrogens from fetal sulfated precursors. The placenta lacks 16-α hydroxylase. All oestriol produced during pregnancy arises from 16-α hydroxylated fetal precursors.

Progesterone

The corpus luteum of the ovary supplies progesterone until about 10 weeks of gestation. This supports pregnancy until placental progesterone production takes over in weeks 7–9 of gestation. Levels of 17α-hydroxyprogesterone produced by the corpus luteum rise in early pregnancy but fall by the 10th week of gestation. After that time, placental production of progesterone dominates the maternal system and the placenta exhibits almost no 17α-hydroxylase activity.

Unlike other steroid-producing glands, the placenta lacks the enzymes to form cholesterol from acetate; therefore, progesterone produced by syncytiotrophoblast cells is dependent on maternal cholesterol. hCG produced by the placenta supports the synthesis and secretion of progesterone within the placenta. Oestrogens may also promote progesterone production by stimulating cholesterol uptake by the placenta and placental enzymatic conversion of cholesterol to pregnenolone. As a result, very large amounts of progesterone are produced and secreted into the maternal bloodstream. This progesterone is active locally within the uterus, where it maintains the decidual lining of the uterus and relaxes the smooth muscle cells of the myometrium. It also has peripheral effects upon vascular smooth muscle and other organs that must adapt to the demands of pregnancy (Chapter 21).

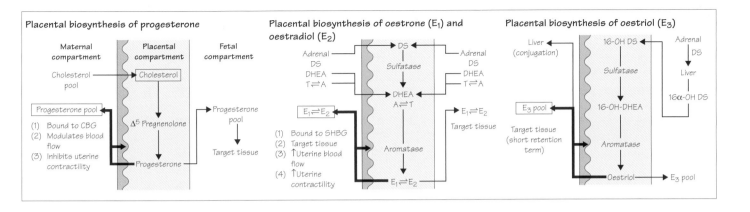

Placental biosynthesis of progesterone

Placental biosynthesis of oestrone (E_1) and oestradiol (E_2)

Placental biosynthesis of oestriol (E_3)

Oestrogens

The placenta can efficiently aromatize androgen precursors to oestrogens because it expresses abundant amounts of the enzyme aromatase. All three of the major oestrogens, oestradiol (E_2), oestrone (E_1) and oestriol (E_3) are produced in the placenta. The androgen precursors for each arise from different sources. Because placental aromatase is so abundant, it is not rate-limiting. Therefore, the relative amounts of each oestrogen produced are determined by the amounts of substrate delivered to the placenta. The **major androgen precursor for placental oestrogen production is dehydroepiandrosterone sulfate (DHEA-S)**. DHEA-S is an adrenal androgen and the majority supplied to the placenta originates in the maternal adrenal gland. In the placenta, DHEA-S is converted to DHEA by the abundant placental sulfate-cleaving enzyme, sulfatase. Maternal DHEA is then converted to androstenedione, then testosterone and finally to oestrone and oestradiol (Chapter 3). A very small amount of fetal DHEA-S is also utilized by the placenta to produce oestrone and oestradiol. **The majority of fetal DHEA-S, however, is converted to oestriol in the placenta**. To accomplish this, most of the fetal DHEA-S first undergoes 16-hydroxylation in the fetal liver. When the fetal 16-OH-DHEA-S reaches the placenta, the placental sulfatase cleaves the sulfate side chain. 16α-OH DHEA is further metabolized and aromatized within the placenta to oestriol. Oestriol, which is not produced by the human ovary, is a relatively weak oestrogen, but when produced at the high levels seen in pregnancy it can have dramatic oestrogenic effects. The amount of oestriol produced by the placenta far exceeds that of oestrone and oestradiol, making **placental oestriol of fetal origin the major placental oestrogen**.

Like progesterone, most of the oestrogen produced by the placenta is found in the maternal compartment (uterus and bloodstream). Unlike its other oestrogenic activities, oestriol appears to be as effective as oestradiol and oestrone in increasing uteroplacental blood flow. Its relatively weak oestrogenic effects on other organ systems make it highly effective in this single important pregnancy function. Its unique production from a fetal substrate also permits fetal regulation of uteroplacental blood flow. Uteroplacental blood flow is an important determinant of fetal growth and well-being.

Fetal adrenal physiology

By about 9 weeks of gestation, the fetal adrenal gland has developed an inner fetal zone and a very thin outer definitive zone. The latter will develop into the adrenal cortex in the adult. Approximately 80% of the gland is composed of the inner fetal zone. The fetal adrenal gland functions independently of ACTH until nearly 15–16 weeks of gestation. During this pre-ACTH phase, the fetal adrenal is thought to respond to hCG. After this time, it is controlled by ACTH secreted by the fetal pituitary gland. The fetal adrenal gland increases in size until about 24 weeks of gestation. It undergoes another impressive growth spurt at 34–35 weeks. 3β-hydroxysteroid dehydrogenase activity is limited in the fetal zone and therefore its major secretory products are DHEA and DHEA-S. These serve as the major substrates for circulating maternal oestrogens. In fact, circulating maternal oestrogen levels reflect the size of the fetal adrenal. Fetal ACTH control of its adrenals is assured by the presence of high levels of oestrogen during pregnancy. Placental oestrogens activate placental 11β-hydroxysteroid dehydrogenase. This in turn metabolizes maternal cortisol, allowing little to reach the fetal circulation.

Maternal adrenal function and salt metabolism

During pregnancy, the zona fasciculata of the maternal adrenal gland increases in size at the expense of the other adrenal cortical zones. In response, maternal glucocorticoid secretion increases, with significant elevations in maternal levels of circulating cortisol. Elevated oestrogen levels also drive an increase in the production of cortisol binding globulin. Still, an increase in the level of circulating free cortisol accompanies the increase in total cortisol. An increase in maternal plasma renin activity and angiotensinogen production results in an increase in plasma aldosterone levels during pregnancy. This results in elevated sodium retention and is partially responsible for the notable increase in maternal vascular volume.

Maternal physiological adaptations to pregnancy

Fetal initiatives

	Maternal response
Volume support	Volume expansion
	Vasodilatation
Nutrition	↑Respiration
	Peripheral insulin resistance
	↑Mineral absorption
Waste clearance	↑Renal glomerular filtration
	Hepatocellular stimulation
Pregnancy maintenance/ maturation	Uterine quiescence
	Immunological sequestration

Maternal physiology must adapt in response to a series of demands attendant to pregnancy. The pregnant woman needs to increase her circulating blood volume to supply nutrients to the fetus and to support amniotic fluid production. She must meet fetal and placental nutritional demands for glucose, amino acids and oxygen. She must clear fetal waste products and protect her pregnancy from systemic perturbations, including starvation or medication ingestion. The maternal system must adapt to allow for the timely onset of labour and for the protection of the mother from cardiovascular insults at the time of delivery. It must also prepare to support nourishment of the infant post-delivery. All maternal organ systems are affected to some degree.

Cardiovascular system

During the first two trimesters of pregnancy, maternal circulating blood volume increases 40% (3500 cm^3 expands to 5000 cm^3). This results from enhancements in the renin–angiotensin system. Placental oestrogen increases hepatic production of angiotensinogen, and oestrogen and progesterone together increase renal production of the proteolytic enzyme, renin. Renin cleaves angiotensinogen to form angiotensin I, which is converted into angiotensin II (AII) in the lung and elsewhere. The increased amounts of AII act on the zona glomerulosa of the adrenal gland to increase aldosterone production. Aldosterone promotes volume expansion through sodium and water retention. Oxygen-carrying capacity must be maintained in the presence of this increase in circulating blood volume. Iron absorption increases to meet the demand for increased haemoglobin during the volume expansion.

A loss of peripheral vascular responsiveness to AII accompanies the increase in circulating blood volume. AII is a potent vasoconstrictor and loss of AII responsivity results in a drop in maternal blood pressure during the early second trimester. This relative hypotension is seen in most pregnant women despite elevated AII levels. Maternal blood pressures will slowly rise to prepregnancy levels by the third trimester. Progesterone promotes overall smooth muscle relaxation and is thereby partially responsible for alterations in maternal blood pressure.

Respiratory system

An increase in tidal volume, minute ventilatory volume and minute O_2 uptake develop in pregnant women. These changes allow for increased oxygen delivery to the fetus and the periphery. They also result in a mild maternal respiratory alkalosis that is compensated for by increased renal bicarbonate excretion. Progesterone may be responsible for many of these changes. Fetal haemoglobin binds O_2 at a lower partial pressure than maternal adult haemoglobin. This favours the transfer of O_2 from mother to fetus within the placenta.

Many pregnant women have the sensation of shortness of breath in the absence of pathology. The reasons for this remain unclear.

Kidney and urinary tract

Maternal glomerular filtration rate (GFR) and renal plasma flow (RPF) begin to increase in early pregnancy. By midpregnancy, maternal GFR has increased by as much as 50%; it remains elevated throughout gestation. In contrast, maternal RPF begins to decrease in the third trimester. As a result, the renal filtration fraction increases during the last third of pregnancy. Because of the increased GFR, serum creatinine and urea are lower in pregnancy than in the non-pregnant state. Creatinine clearance is increased.

A 60–70% increase in the filtered load of sodium also accompanies the increased GFR. Progesterone appears to cause some sodium wastage by interfering with normal sodium resorption in the proximal renal tubule. In response, aldosterone increases proportionately to levels that are 2–3 times normal.

The relatively fixed renal tubular reabsorptive capacity, in combination with an increased GFR, causes a decrease in the reabsorption of glucose from the proximal tubule of the pregnant woman's kidney. Glucose is therefore detectable in the urine of about 15% of normal pregnant women. Still, any pregnant woman exhibiting glycosuria should be evaluated for diabetes.

The volume of urine contained in the renal pelves and ureters can double in the latter half of pregnancy. The renal collecting system dilates during pregnancy due to mechanical obstruction by the pregnant uterus combined with the relaxing effects of progesterone upon smooth muscle. This dilatation decreases the speed of urine passage through the renal system and increases the maternal risk of developing acute kidney infections.

Gastrointestinal tract and metabolism

Pregnancy is a potentially diabetogenic state. It is a state of relative hyperinsulinism with peripheral insulin resistance. The high maternal levels of oestrogen, progesterone and placental lactogen (hPL) cause hypertrophy, hyperplasia and hypersecretion of insulin by the beta islet cells of the pancreas. Still, many pregnant women show prolonged hyperglycaemia after meals. In addition, most pregnant women exhibit: (i) exaggerated insulin release in response to glucose infusion, (ii) reduced peripheral uptake of glucose, and (iii) suppressed glucagon secretion. Taken together, these traits characterize insulin resistance. The mechanism(s) for insulin resistance are not well understood. The growth hormone-like activity of hPL may be responsible. In addition, hPL may also promote lipolysis and liberation of free fatty acids that facilitates tissue resistance to insulin. These metabolic changes ensure a continuous supply of glucose for transfer to the fetus but produce an 'accelerated starvation' profile in the fasted pregnant woman. Fasted pregnant women are relatively hypoglycaemic and have higher circulating free fatty acids, triglycerides and cholesterol. Prolonged fasting or persistent vomiting in pregnant women can rapidly lead to ketonaemia.

High maternal levels of circulating oestrogens increase the synthesis of hepatic proteins. These include procoagulants, bile acids and multiple hormone binding proteins. The procoagulants most markedly elevated are Factors I (fibrinogen), VII, VIII, IX and X. The higher circulating concentrations of clotting cascade proteins protect the mother from excessive blood loss at the time of delivery; however, they also predispose pregnant and postpartum women to an increased risk for venous thrombosis and embolism. Oestrogens also stimulate the cytochrome P450 oxidative pathway in the liver. This increases the production of steroid precursors and can dramatically alter drug metabolism. (The latter effect necessitates careful monitoring of the maternal plasma drug levels of many commonly used therapeutics. Most notable are the anticonvulsants and antibiotics.)

The calcium requirements of the developing fetal and neonatal skeleton produce a profound maternal calcium stress during pregnancy and lactation. Maternal plasma parathyroid hormone (PTH) concentrations rise despite a minimal decrease in circulating free calcium. Intestinal absorption of calcium is enhanced by an increase in circulating 1,25-dihydroxyvitamin D_3, the active metabolite of vitamin D. 1,25-$(OH)_2$-D_3 increases for two reasons: (i) PTH increases the hepatic synthesis of 25-(OH)-D_3, and (ii) the activity of 1α-hydroxylase increases in pregnancy. In non-pregnant women and men, conversion of 25-(OH)-D_3 to the 1,25 active form is limited by the activity of 1α-hydroxylase, the final converting enzyme in D_3 metabolism. 1α-hydroxylase is typically present only in the kidney but, in pregnancy, it is produced by both the decidua and placenta. This ensures an adequate amount of active D_3 to optimize dietary calcium absorption during pregnancy. If dietary calcium intake is adequate, minimal mobilization of maternal bone calcium occurs. If it is not, fetal and neonatal skeletal mineralization will proceed at the expense of maternal bone density.

Progesterone relaxes smooth muscle and thereby affects all parts of the gastrointestinal (GI) tract during pregnancy. Gastric emptying is delayed, as is movement of digested material along the remainder of the tract. Gallbladder emptying is slower and bile tends to sludge in the bile duct and common duct. Minor disorders of the GI tract are very common in pregnancy. These include nausea, vomiting, constipation and heartburn.

Haematological system

Pregnant women are mildly anaemic. Maternal haemoglobin production and total red blood cell mass increases during pregnancy in response to elevated erythropoietin production. Maternal vascular volume increases to a greater extent. The result is a mild maternal dilutional anaemia that protects the mother from excess haemoglobin loss at delivery. The iron requirements of normal pregnancy must satisfy both maternal and fetal red cell production requirements and total about 1.0 g. Most is needed during the second half of pregnancy. The amount of iron absorbed from the diet alone, as well as any mobilized from maternal stores, may be insufficient to meet the demand.

Pregnant women develop a modest leucocytosis that can become quite marked during labour and postpartum. The aetiology of the mild leucocytosis of early pregnancy is unclear. That seen during labour, however, resembles the leucocytosis associated with strenuous exercise, during which previously sequestered white cells re-enter the active circulation.

Pregnant women are hypercoagulable. Increased coagulability develops because of the increased procoagulant synthesis in the liver. Up to 8% of women will develop a mild thrombocytopenia (<150 000 platelets/mL). This typically does not result in a bleeding diathesis. The mechanism by which the thrombocytopenia develops is unknown.

Thyroid gland

The elevated circulating levels of oestrogen in the pregnant woman stimulate hepatic protein synthesis, including the production of thyroid-binding globulin (TBG). Pregnant women have higher levels of TBG, total T_3 and T_4, but normal amounts of free T_3 and T_4.

Immune system

The fetus represents a hemi-allograft in a typically immunocompetent host. Graft rejection usually does not occur. Alterations in maternal immune responsivity favouring fetal tolerance include a decrease in general cellular immunity. In addition, the placenta does not express classical transplantation antigens, including major histocompatibility complex (MHC) class II and most MHC class I products. Altered maternal immune responsivity during pregnancy results in a higher attack rate and more severe or prolonged disease upon exposure to certain viral pathogens (e.g. varicella/chicken pox).

Skin

Circulating melanotrophic hormone (MSH) is increased during pregnancy as a result of the increased production of the precursor molecule POM-C (Chapter 19). MSH causes darkening on the skin across the cheeks (chloasma or pregnancy mask) and darkening of the linea alba, the slightly pigmented line on the skin that runs from the navel to the pubis. Hair may also appear to fall out in clumps because of synchronization of hair follicle growth cycles during pregnancy.

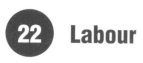
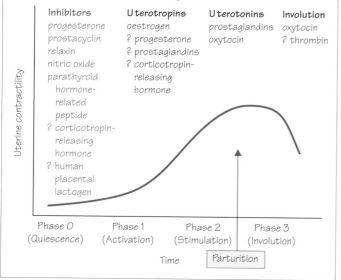

Phases of labour and their regulation

Inhibitors	Uterotropins	Uterotonins	Involution
progesterone	oestrogen	prostaglandins	oxytocin
prostacyclin	? progesterone	oxytocin	? thrombin
relaxin	? prostaglandins		
nitric oxide	? corticotropin-		
parathyroid	releasing		
hormone-	hormone		
related			
peptide			
? corticotropin-			
releasing			
hormone			
? human			
placental			
lactogen			

Phase 0 (Quiescence) Phase 1 (Activation) Phase 2 (Stimulation) Phase 3 (Involution)

Time · Parturition

Labour is the process by which the fetus and its supporting placenta and membranes pass from the uterus to the outside world. **It is defined as regular uterine contractions that result in thinning and dilatation of the cervix so that the products of conception can pass out of the uterus.** Labour involves three key processes: (i) a switch in myometrial activity, from a longer-lasting, low-frequency irregular contraction pattern called 'contractures' to the frequent, high-intensity, regular pattern known as 'contractions'; (ii) softening and dilatation of the cervix; and (iii) rupture of the fetal membranes. Although labour may first become apparent with the isolated appearance of any of these three elements, the physiological events that produce them typically occur simultaneously.

Phases of labour

It is useful to consider labour as a series of four physiological phases, characterized by the release of the myometrium from the inhibitory effects of pregnancy and the activation of stimulants of myometrial contractility. Phase 0 comprises the majority of pregnancy. During this phase, the uterus is maintained in a state of quiescence by one or more inhibitors of contractility. Candidate inhibitors include progesterone, prostacyclin, nitric oxide, parathyroid hormone-related peptide (PTHrP), calcitonin gene-related peptide, relaxin, adrenomedullin and vasoactive intestinal peptide (VIP). Near the end of a normal pregnancy, the uterus undergoes the process of activation (Phase 1). During activation, a number of contraction-associated proteins increase under the influence of oestrogen. These proteins include myometrial receptors for prostaglandins and oxytocin, membranous ion channels and connexin-43, a key component of gap junctions. The increase in myometrial gap junctions during activation will electrically couple adjacent myometrial cells and maximize the coordination of contraction waves that move from the uterine fundus to the cervix. Phase 2 of labour is called stimulation. During stimulation, oxytocin and stimulatory prostaglandins (PGs) such as PGE_2 and $PGF_{2\alpha}$ can induce contractions in the previously primed uterus. The cervix dilates. The fetus, membranes and

placenta are expelled from the uterus in a process called parturition. Phase 3 of labour follows parturition and is called involution. During involution, sustained contraction of the uterus promotes necessary haemostasis and eventually reduces the massively enlarged postpartum uterus to a size only slightly larger than its prepregnant state.

Initiation of labour

The average human gestation lasts 280 days (40 weeks) from the beginning of the last menstrual period. Exactly what triggers human labour is unknown. Still, like other species that bear live young, the fetoplacental unit appears to control at what point in gestation labour will occur while maternal signals determine the time of day that it will start. The mechanisms used by the fetoplacental unit to initiate labour vary from species to species. Humans mimic the mechanisms used by other primates much more closely than those used by more distantly related mammals.

Sheep and rodents rely on progesterone withdrawal for labour initiation. In stark contrast, the initiation of labour in primates involves an increase in placental oestrogen synthesis. It appears that this oestrogen must be produced by the placenta, because systemic infusion of oestrogen does not induce labour at term. Rather, infused androstenedione will induce contractions and this effect can be blocked by inhibiting aromatase activity. Placental aromatase activity (Chapters 3 and 19) increases at term. This is accompanied by an increase in production of adrenal androgen precursors (e.g. androstenedione) by the fetus. Both support increased placental oestrogen production.

The stimulus for the increase in fetal adrenal androgen production near term is not known. It does not appear to arise from the fetal hypothalamus (corticotrophin-releasing factor, CRH) or pituitary adrenocorticotrophic hormone (ACTH) because absence of appropriate brain formation in anencephalic fetuses does not prolong pregnancy. Rather, the stimulus is likely to be placental. Placental CRH is an excellent candidate. Placental CRH is biochemically identical to maternal and fetal hypothalamic CRH but differs in its regulation. Glucocorticoids exert negative feedback on the synthesis and release of hypothalamic CRH, but stimulate placental CRH. Placental CRH appears to stimulate fetal ACTH production and fetal adrenal steroid synthesis (e.g. androstenedione production). It may also have local effects within the uterus, fostering placental vasodilatation, prostaglandin production and myometrial contractility.

In all species, an increase in prostaglandin synthesis by the decidua and the fetal membranes constitutes the final common pathway in labour. Human uterine tissues are selectively enriched with arachidonic acid, an essential fatty acid that is the obligate precursor of those prostaglandins most important in labour: PGE and $PGF_{2\alpha}$. Both cyclo-oxygenase enzymes, COX-1 and COX-2, are expressed in the uterus. COX-2, the inducible form of the enzyme, appears to be sensitive to glucocorticoid induction. Evidence for the role of prostaglandins in labour includes observations that: (i) the concentrations of PGs in amniotic fluid, maternal plasma and maternal urine are increased just prior to the onset of labour; (ii) administration of PGs at any stage of pregnancy has the capacity to initiate labour; (iii) PGs can induce cervical ripening and uterine contractions; (iv) PGs increase myometrial sensitivity to oxytocin; and (v) inhibitors of PG synthesis can suppress

Proposed mechanisms of labour induction at term

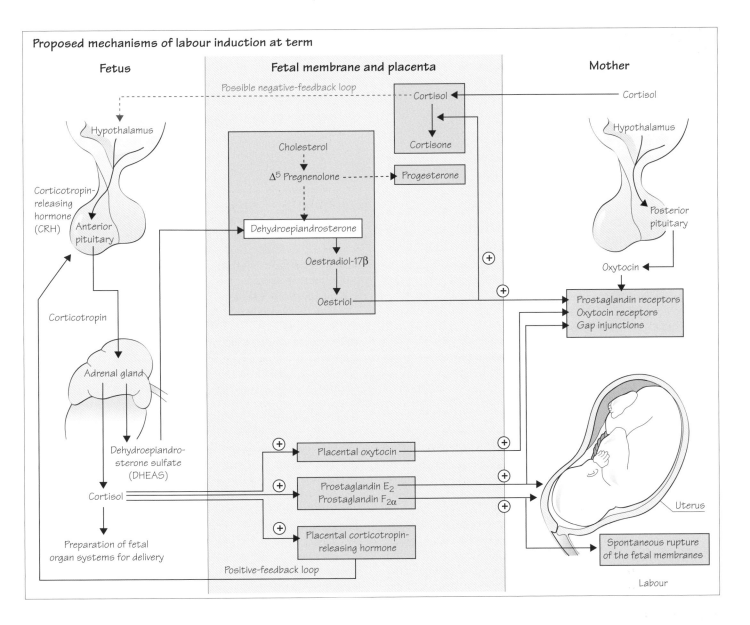

contractions and prolong pregnancy (e.g. the COX inhibitor, indomethacin).

Like other smooth muscle cells, myometrial cells are triggered to contract by a rise in intracellular calcium (Ca^{2+}). Prostaglandins raise intracellular Ca^{2+} by increasing Ca^{2+} influx across the cell membranes, by stimulating calcium release from intracellular stores and by enhancing myometrial gap junction formation.

Oxytocin, a posterior pituitary hormone, plays an important role in labour. Oxytocin acts through its membrane receptor on myometrial cells to activate members of the G-protein subfamily. These, in turn, activate phospholipase C and inositol triphosphate, causing a release of intracellular Ca^{2+}. Oxytocin appears to play a role in the maternal control of the time of day that labour will start. Several days to weeks before the onset of recognizable labour, myometrial activity switches away from contractures to contractions. This switch invariably occurs when the lights go off in the animal's environment and ensures that delivery will occur when the mother is safely at rest away from

predators. Nocturnally active animals will thus deliver during the day and vice versa. This circadian rhythm of uterine activity is accompanied by an increase in both circulating oxytocin and myometrial oxytocin receptors.

Oxytocin also plays an important role in promoting expulsion of the fetus from the uterus after the cervix is fully dilated. In fact, the oxytocin concentrations in the maternal circulation do not begin to rise until the expulsive stage of labour begins. Still, the gradual increase in the concentrations of oxytocin receptor in the myometrium during the second half of pregnancy may allow for lower concentrations of oxytocin to effect myometrial contractions prior to the onset of expulsion. Oxytocin can induce prostaglandin production and gap junction formation within the uterus, suggesting that it may act in synergy with other factors to initiate labour. To this point, oxytocin can be used clinically to induce and to stimulate labour. The fetus, placenta and fetal membranes all make oxytocin that is selectively secreted toward the maternal compartment.

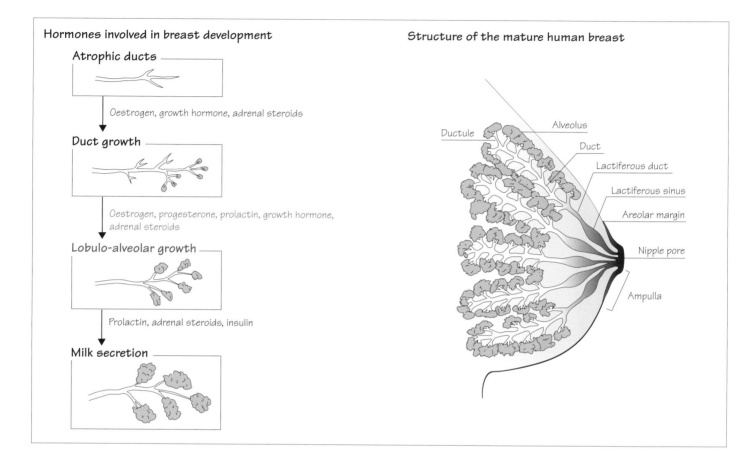

Hormones involved in breast development

Atrophic ducts

↓ Oestrogen, growth hormone, adrenal steroids

Duct growth

↓ Oestrogen, progesterone, prolactin, growth hormone, adrenal steroids

Lobulo-alveolar growth

↓ Prolactin, adrenal steroids, insulin

Milk secretion

Structure of the mature human breast

Ductule · Alveolus · Duct · Lactiferous duct · Lactiferous sinus · Areolar margin · Nipple pore · Ampulla

Development of the breast

The human mammary gland is derived from ectoderm. It is first visible in the 4-week embryo as a bud or nodule of epithelial tissue appearing along a line known as the milk crest. In the more developed embryo, this crest extends from the midaxilla to the inguinal region and may be the site of supernumerary breasts or nipples in the adult. The rudimentary epithelial nodule first becomes buried in embryonic mesenchyme, where it undergoes further differentiation, apparently under the influence of paracrine signals from the mesenchyme. Secondary epithelial buds form cellular cords that elongate, bifurcate and cavitate. These cords become the excretory and lactiferous ducts of the mammary gland.

The human mammary gland is a compound tuboalveolar structure composed of 15–25 irregular lobes radiating out from the nipple. Individual lobes are embedded in adipose tissue and separated by dense layers of connective tissue. Each lobe is further subdivided into lobules, connected to the nipple by lactiferous ducts. The lactiferous ducts are lined by a stratified squamous epithelium. Loose connective tissue (stroma) surrounds the lactiferous ducts and permits their ready distension during lactation.

At birth, the breast is rudimentary and consists almost entirely of lactiferous ducts. Although it may secrete a few drops of milk, called 'witch's milk', this secretory function is short-lived and the breast quickly becomes quiescent until puberty. At puberty, ovarian oestrogens stimulate the lactiferous duct system to grow. After menarche, exposure to cyclic progesterone induces further ductal growth and development of rudimentary lobules at the ends of the ducts. Ductal epithelium remains sensitive to oestrogen stimulation throughout a woman's reproductive years; stromal tissue remains sensitive to progesterone stimulation. The breasts continue to grow for several years after menarche as the lactiferous ducts progressively subdivide, elongate and hollow out, and adipose tissue accumulates. However, lobular development will not go beyond a rudimentary stage in the absence of pregnancy.

At the beginning of pregnancy there is rapid growth and branching of the terminal portions of the rudimentary lobules. Vascularity increases dramatically. The pregnant woman often perceives these two changes as a 'tingling' or 'tension' in her breasts. This may begin shortly after conception and last throughout the first trimester. At about 8 menstrual weeks of pregnancy, true alveolar differentiation begins. True glandular acini appear as hollow alveoli lined with a single layer of myoepithelial cells. The highly branched myoepithelial cells form a loose network surrounding the alveoli. The alveoli connect to the larger lactiferous ducts through intralobular ducts. Alveolar secretion begins in the second trimester of pregnancy. By the third trimester, an immunoglobulin-rich secretion is seen distending the alveoli.

While the role of ovarian steroids in breast development is clearly clinically established (prepubertal gonadal failure is associated with absence of breast development), animal models suggest that other hormones may also be involved in human breast development. Insulin exposure causes multiplication of epithelial cells and formation of lobuloalveolar architecture. Complete cytological and functional differentiation of the epithelial cells lining the alveoli requires exposure to cortisol, insulin and prolactin. Receptors for growth factors such as insulin-like growth factor I (IGF-I) and epidermal growth factor (EGF) have been demonstrated on human mammary cells, suggesting an important role for their ligands in breast development and function.

Milk formation

Milk has more than 100 constituents. It is basically an emulsion of fat in a liquid phase that is isotonic with plasma. Mature human milk contains 3–5% fat, 1% protein, 7% lactose and 0.2% minerals, and delivers 60–75 kcal/dL. The principal class of human milk lipids is triglycerides, of which palmitic and oleic acids are the most abundant. The main proteins in human milk are casein, α-lactalbumin, lactoferrin, immunoglobulin A, lysozyme and albumin. Casein and α-lactalbumin are specific milk proteins; α-lactalbumin is part of the enzyme complex lactose synthetase. Lactose is the primary sugar in human milk. Free amino acids, urea, creatinine and creatine are also present. Minerals include sodium, potassium, calcium, magnesium, phosphorus and chloride. As the composition of human breast milk continues to be studied, several peptide hormones, including EGF, transforming growth factor α (TGF-α), somatostatin and IGF-I and IGF-II have also been identified. The first milk secreted after delivery is called colostrum. It contains a higher protein content (largely immunoglobulins) and lower sugar content than subsequent secretions.

The alveolar epithelial cells that make milk are polarized, highly differentiated cells whose function is to accumulate, synthesize, package and export the components of milk. **At least four transcellular pathways** are required for appropriate **milk formation** within the alveolus of the breast. The first involves **secretion of monovalent cations and water**. Water is drawn across the alveolar cell by a concentration gradient generated by specific milk sugars; ions follow an electrochemical gradient. The second involves **receptor-mediated transport of immunoglobulins**. Immunoglobulin A enters the epithelial cell after binding to its receptor, becomes internalized and is transported either to the Golgi apparatus or the apical membrane of the cell for secretion. The third pathway involves the **synthesis and transport of milk lipids**, which are synthesized in the cytoplasm and smooth endoplasmic reticulum. They then aggregate into droplets that coalesce to form larger fat globules. These are discharged from the apical part of the cell into the alveolar lumen. The final pathway involves **exocytosis of secretory vesicles containing specific milk proteins, calcium, phosphate, citrate and lactose**. These vesicles form in the Golgi apparatus. Here, casein, the specific milk protein, forms micelles with calcium and phosphate. The Golgi is impermeable to lactose. Because lactose is an osmotically active sugar, water is drawn into the Golgi and lactose content thereby determines the milk's liquid volume. A fifth pathway is required for milk formation: it is not transcellular, but paracellular. Immunoglobulins, such as IgA, plasma proteins and leukocytes can move between alveolar cells that have lost their tight junctions.

Regulation of milk production

Regulation of the quantity and content of breast milk is largely under hormonal control, with **prolactin** being the most important regulatory hormone in humans, although its actions require synergism with several others. Prolactin concentrations in the plasma rise steadily throughout pregnancy, from less than 20 ng/mL to over 200 ng/mL at term

(Chapter 19). In breastfeeding women, basal serum prolactin levels remain elevated for about 4–6 weeks postpartum, then fall to non-pregnant levels despite continued lactation. For about the next 2 months, suckling causes spikes of prolactin release. Even with production of a litre or more of breast milk per day, this reflex is also gradually lost.

The pivotal role of prolactin in the initiation of breastfeeding was established by blocking secretion of the hormone from the pituitary using the dopamine agonist, bromocriptine. When bromocriptine is given to women shortly after delivery, prolactin levels drop precipitously to non-pregnant levels. Breast engorgement and lactation never occur. Oestrogens can also be used to suppress lactation immediately postpartum, but they work through a different mechanism. After oestrogen administration, prolactin levels remain quite elevated, but no milk is formed. Thus oestrogens inhibit the action of prolactin on the breast, which is probably why lactation does not occur before delivery. With delivery of the placenta, the source of the large amount of circulating oestrogen is removed. Circulating oestrogens drop precipitously and breast milk begins to form within 24–48 h. Bromocriptine administered later in the postpartum period also inhibits lactation, but only until the process no longer depends on prolactin.

Prolactin has several actions at the cellular level. It stimulates the synthesis of β-lactoglobulin and casein in breast tissue primed by insulin and cortisol. It stabilizes casein mRNA, prolonging its half-life eight-fold. Prolactin stimulates milk fat synthesis, and may be involved in sodium transport in mammary tissue. Interestingly, and unlike other polypeptide hormones, prolactin binding to its receptor does not stimulate adenylate cyclase activity.

The lactation reflex

Although prolactin is responsible for initiating milk production, milk delivery to the infant and lactation maintenance depend on mechanical stimulation of the nipple. The suckling stimulus is known as **milk ejection** or **letdown**. Although suckling is the major stimulus for milk letdown, the reflex can be conditioned. The cry or sight of an infant and preparation of the breast for nursing may cause letdown, while pain, embarrassment and alcohol can inhibit it.

The suckling reflex is initiated when sensory impulses originating in the nipple enter the spinal cord through its dorsal roots. A multisynaptic neural pathway ascends to the magnocellular supraoptic and paraventricular nuclei of the hypothalamus via activin-containing neurons in the nucleus solitarius tract. Impulse recognition results in episodic **oxytocin** release from the posterior pituitary. Oxytocin then stimulates the myoepithelial cells lining the milk ducts to contract, thereby causing milk 'ejection'.

A large surge in prolactin release is temporally associated with the episodic oxytocin release induced by nursing, but this surge will occur independently of the oxytocin changes. This transient pulse of prolactin induces milk formation for the next feeding. Smoking can inhibit this prolactin surge and cause a decrease in milk production.

The suckling reflex also affects the activity of the gonadotrophin-releasing hormone (GnRH) pulse generator. Suckling inhibits gonadotropin release and ovulation does not typically occur. The effectiveness of lactation in suppressing gonadal function is directly related to the frequency and duration of nursing. Among the !Kung hunter-gatherers in Africa, the average interval between births is 44 months in spite of early postpartum resumption of coitus and lack of contraception. Mothers nurse about every 15 min and children are in immediate proximity to their mothers all day and night for 2 years or more.

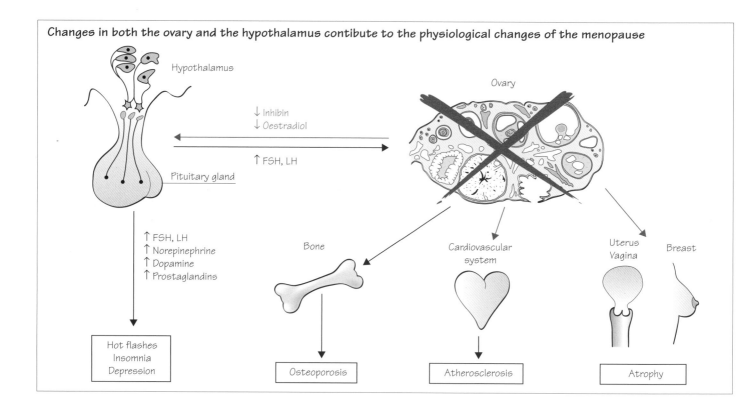

Changes in both the ovary and the hypothalamus contibute to the physiological changes of the menopause

Menopause is a normal stage of life. Its health consequences have only become apparent as life expectancy has increased well beyond the 6th decade of life for women. It is estimated that women living in developed countries will live at least one-third of their lives after menopause. Functionally, menopause may be considered an '**oestrogen withdrawal syndrome**'. It is recognizable by the loss of menses and, for most women, by the appearance of signs and symptoms such as hot flashes, insomnia, vaginal atrophy, decreased breast size and reduced skin elasticity. Osteoporosis and cardiovascular disease represent longer-term consequences of oestrogen deficiency. Both are more indolent and less predictable than the early signs and symptoms of menopause.

Physiology of menopause

The postmenopausal ovary is small and essentially devoid of follicles. The appearance of the postmenopausal ovary, coupled with the observation that oophorectomy is associated with menopausal symptoms, led to the original theory that follicular depletion was responsible for menopause. More recent evidence suggests that menopause has origins in both the central nervous system and the ovary. In addition, men appear to experience a similar, albeit later and more subtle change, called andropause. Both changes can be referred to as 'gonopause' and associated mechanisms in the central nervous system and gonads seem to be quite extensive and to reflect the general aging process.

Fertility decreases dramatically in women beginning at about age 35 but accelerating after the age of 40. The accelerated fall after 40 may be the first sign of impending ovarian failure. Although ovarian follicles remain visible on ultrasound, attempts at artificial induction of ovulation with injected gonadotropins are largely unsuccessful after about age 45 years. This suggests that a physiological defect develops within the oocytes or follicles prior to their depletion. About 3–4 years before menopause is apparent, serum follicle-stimulating hormone (FSH) levels begin to rise subtly and ovarian oestrogen, inhibin and progesterone production falls. Menstrual cycle length tends to decrease as the follicular phase progressively shortens. Ultimately, ovulation and menstruation cease entirely. The age of onset of menopause has changed very little over time—even the ancient Greeks mention the age of 50 as typical. Age of menopause is affected by multiple factors. Maternal menopausal age is predictive of a daughter's menopausal age. Age of menarche does not affect age of menopause. Most agree that race and parity have no effect. Smokers enter menopause at an earlier age than non-smokers.

Although ovarian failure is a major component of menopause, functional alterations occur at the level of the pituitary as well. Changes arise in the intrinsic rhythms, which control sleep and the neuroendocrine axes. Such changes in the circadian oscillator lead to diminished nocturnal melatonin secretion and altered sleep, decreased responsiveness of the gonadotropin axis to steroid feedback and decreased adrenal steroid production. Aging is also associated with a more general decline in central dopaminergic and noradrenergic neuronal function. Oestrogen deficiency further exacerbates the dopamine deficiency by increasing the ratio of norepinephrine to dopamine.

During menopause, the decrease in ovarian oestrogen and inhibin production reduces negative feedback signals to the pituitary and hypothalamus and results in a progressive rise in gonadotropin levels.

Because inhibin acts exclusively to regulate FSH (Chapter 2), FSH levels rise disproportionately to luteinizing hormone (LH) levels. **When in doubt, persistent elevation of serum FSH levels confirms the diagnosis of menopause.** Although ovarian oestrogen production essentially ceases, the ovary continues to make the androgens testosterone and androstenedione. Most of this steroid biosynthesis occurs in the hilar cells of the medulla of the gland and very little occurs in the stroma. Hilar cells share a common embryological origin with testicular Leydig cells, the main androgen-secreting cells in the male (Chapter 9).

Although ovarian oestrogen production ceases at menopause, postmenopausal women are not completely oestrogen deficient. Peripheral tissues such as fat, liver and kidney express the enzyme aromatase and can convert circulating androgens to oestrogens. The major difference between direct ovarian oestrogen secretion and peripheral conversion is that most of the oestrogen produced by the latter process is oestrone. Oestrone is the oestrogen produced from aromatization of androstenedione, the major androgen secreted by the postmenopausal ovary and adrenal gland (Chapter 3). Oestrone is a very weak oestrogen compared to oestradiol. In the typical concentrations found in postmenopausal women, oestrone does not provide protection against the long-term consequences of oestrogen deficiency. Obese postmenopausal women are protected from this. Fat is a particularly rich source of aromatase activity and obese postmenopausal women can produce substantial amounts of oestrone. These high quantities of endogenous oestrone provide some protection against the risk of menopausal vasomotor symptoms and osteoporosis but at a cost. Prolonged exposure of the endometrium to oestrogen stimulation that is unopposed by postovulatory progesterone will increase the risk for the development of endometrial hyperplasia and carcinoma (Chapter 42). The endometrium is never converted from proliferative physiology to secretory morphology and this unregulated growth favours neoplastic change. A similar risk of endometrial stimulation is present in women receiving oestrogen alone for postmenopausal hormone replacement.

Signs and symptoms
Hot flashes
Hot flashes or flushes occur in about 75% of menopausal women. Nocturnal hot flashes often wake a woman from sleep and may produce significant sleep deprivation or insomnia. During a hot flash most women note a sensation of pressure in their head followed by a flush of heat or burning. This sensation begins on the head or neck area and passes over the entire body. Sweating invariably accompanies the flush. While there are profound physiological changes associated with hot flashes, the mechanism by which oestrogen deficiency produces this symptom is not known. The physiological changes include an initial increase in skin conductance and then temperature, a reflection of peripheral vasodilatation. Core body temperature subsequently drops by an average of 0.2°C. Circulating oestrogen levels do not change before or after the flash but LH, cortisol, dehydroepiandrosterone (DHEA), androstenedione and the pro-opiomelanocortin (POM-C)-derived peptides all do. It is believed that the hot flash represents an initial change in central thermoregulation that elicits a number of compensatory mechanisms. These mechanisms transiently raise, but ultimately reduce the core body temperature to the new set point. Central nervous system catecholamines are involved in hypothalamic temperature regulation and the impact of oestrogen deficiency on noradrenergic neuronal function likely plays a role in hot flashes. Some hypothesize that oestrogen deficiency predisposes to vasodilatation within the hypothalamus. This results in an increase in hypothalamic temperature and a response favouring a reduction in the core body temperature.

In addition to hot flashes, most menopausal women experience **vaginal atrophy and changes in their breasts and skin**. Vaginal atrophy can lead to decreased vaginal lubrication. This may be physically uncomfortable, may predispose to urinary tract infections, and may result in dyspareunia during intercourse. These changes are directly related to the loss of oestrogen stimulation in target tissues and can largely be reversed by oestrogen replacement.

Bone changes
Bone loss in women actually begins at about age 30. It accelerates at menopause. The most rapid bone loss occurs in the first 3–4 years after menopause. Bone loss occurs more quickly in women who smoke and in very thin women. African-American race and fluoride treatment of the water supply are associated with a lower incidence of osteoporosis. The most common site of osteoporosis-related fractures is the vertebral body, an effect that may be noted clinically as back pain and the development of a 'dowager's hump'. The upper femur, humerus, ribs and distal forearm are also frequently affected by postmenopausal bone loss. Upper femoral fractures that involve the hip joint may be life-threatening because of an accompanying risk of venous thromboembolic disease.

Osteoporosis resulting from prolonged oestrogen deficiency involves a reduction in the quantity of bone without alterations in its chemical composition. Bone formation by osteoblasts is normal in oestrogen-deficient women but the rate of bone resorption by osteoclasts is increased. Trabecular bone is affected first, followed by cortical bone. Oestrogen appears to antagonize the effects of parathyroid hormone (PTH) on calcium mobilization. This may occur as a direct effect of oestrogen on bone because oestrogen receptors have been found on bone cells in culture.

Cardiovascular changes
Oestrogen receptors are present on blood vessels and oestrogen appears to clinically decrease vascular resistance and increase blood flow. One potential mechanism by which oestrogen may improve blood flow is through its demonstrated ability to decrease the production of endothelin, a potent vasoconstrictor, by vascular endothelium. Oestrogen therapy is also associated with an increase in high-density lipoproteins and decrease in low-density lipoproteins. Despite these mechanistic findings, the results of several recent large population studies have suggested that postmenopausal hormone replacement (HRT) may have untoward cardiovascular effects. These results need to be taken in context with risks and benefits weighed for a particular patient. For instance, one arm of the Women's Health Initiative, which is the largest randomized trial of HRT, showed that use of combinations of oestrogen and progestin in the treatment of postmenopausal women resulted in seven additional cases of heart disease, eight pulmonary emboli, eight strokes and eight additional cases of breast cancer among 10 000 women treated for one year. At the same time, there were six fewer cases of colon cancer and five fewer hip fractures. This resulted in 20 women who were harmed by therapy out of 10 000 undergoing treatment. Alternative medications and delivery systems for postmenopausal hormone replacement are under investigation.

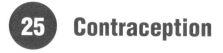

25 Contraception

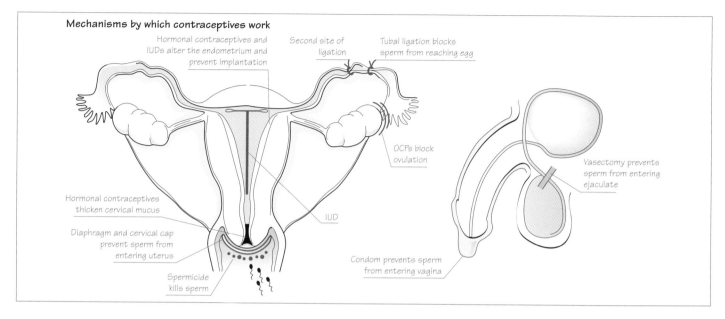

Mechanisms by which contraceptives work

Hormonal contraceptives and IUDs alter the endometrium and prevent implantation

Second site of ligation

Tubal ligation blocks sperm from reaching egg

OCPs block ovulation

Vasectomy prevents sperm from entering ejaculate

Hormonal contraceptives thicken cervical mucus

Diaphragm and cervical cap prevent sperm from entering uterus

IUD

Spermicide kills sperm

Condom prevents sperm from entering vagina

Overview

No form of contraception is perfect. Each has a finite failure rate linked both to the method itself and to the human frailties of the user. Most also have side-effects, some of which can be quite serious. The choice of the right contraceptive for an individual or a couple is a complex decision.

The risk of pregnancy with no contraception is 2–4% for each unprotected act of intercourse, amounting to an overall risk of 85 pregnancies per 100 woman years (equivalent to 100 women using no contraception for 1 year).

'Natural' family planning

Natural family planning or fertility awareness aims to avoid conception by abstention from intercourse during the woman's fertile period. It makes use of a calendar and some indicator of ovulation (basal body temperature measurements, cervical mucus characteristics or commercial ovulation prediction kits) to determine when a woman typically ovulates in her monthly menstrual cycle. Intercourse is avoided during the so-called 'fertile period' at ovulation and for several days before and after. Natural family planning requires a highly motivated couple and the willingness to tolerate some risk of failure. It works best for women with regular menstrual cycles.

The method has no medical side-effects and is accepted by virtually all religions. It has a failure rate of 5–35%, with most populations experiencing rates approaching the higher figure.

Barrier methods

There are three general categories: condom, diaphragm and cervical cap. All three work by preventing spermatozoa from entering the woman's uterus and fertilizing an egg. Barrier methods are good choices for individuals who want to limit contraceptive efficacy to a particular sexual episode. They are readily reversible and can be used in conjunction with timing methods associated with natural family planning. The most serious side-effects of barrier methods occur in individuals with an unknown latex allergy.

Condoms that fit over the man's penis are more widely available than condoms that fit inside the woman's vagina (the female condom). Male condoms may be made from latex rubber, polyurethane or animal intestines; each provides a different 'feel' or sensitivity for the man during intercourse. Female condoms are typically made of polyurethane. An intact condom stops sperm and infectious agents from entering the vagina, and so can prevent transmission of HIV and other sexually transmitted diseases. It must be carefully removed after ejaculation to avoid spilling semen from the condom into the vagina. The failure rates of 3–6% may be improved by using a spermicide (see below).

The **diaphragm** is a soft latex or plastic dome that fits inside the vagina and covers the cervix. Because some sperm may be able to bypass the diaphragm and gain access to the uterus the diaphragm is typically used with a spermicide placed in the dome. Diaphragms should be individually fitted by a health professional and some training is required in their proper insertion and removal. A diaphragm should be left in place for 6–8 h after intercourse, and additional spermicide placed into the vagina if more episodes of intercourse occur before it is removed. Diaphragms partially protect against HIV and other sexually transmitted diseases. Some women develop bladder or vaginal infections during diaphragm use. The failure rate of a properly fitted diaphragm is about 6%; improper fitting or not using a spermicide increases the rate substantially.

Cervical caps are similar to, but smaller than, the diaphragm. They fit tightly over the cervix and must be individually fitted. Cervical caps are not widely available.

Spermicides

These are chemicals that kill sperm by disrupting their outer cell membranes. The most commonly used are nonoxynol-9 and octoxynol-9. Spermicides are available suspended in one of three vehicles: foam, jelly or wax suppositories. They are most effective when used with a barrier method. There are few absolute contraindications to their use. They have an unpleasant taste and can cause an allergy in some users. Spermicide use may cause vaginal inflammation and has been associated with an increase in the transmission of sexually transmitted infections, including HIV. The failure rate of spermicides used alone is 5–15%.

Intrauterine device (IUD)

This is a small T-shaped plastic device that is placed into the uterine cavity. Attached to it is a nylon thread that hangs into the vagina, allowing the user to confirm that it remains in place. An IUD prevents implantation of the fertilized egg by several mechanisms. If it is wrapped with copper, the mineral produces a local inflammatory response in the endometrium and excess prostaglandin production. The copper ion competitively inhibits a number of zinc-requiring processes in sperm activation and endometrium/embryo signalling. If the IUD is impregnated with progestin, the normal proliferative-to-secretory sequence of endometrial maturation is disrupted, creating an intrauterine environment unsatisfactory for implantation.

Historically, certain IUDs have been associated with an increased risk for medical complications and reproductive damage among users who were infected with sexually transmitted pathogens. Modern IUDs are associated with far fewer complications and pose risk only in women actively infected with a pathogen at the time of IUD insertion. Still, many practitioners do not recommend the IUD for women who have not had children or who have multiple sexual partners. Significant non-infectious side-effects include excessive menstrual bleeding, iron-deficiency anaemia, dysmenorrhoea and septic abortion if pregnancy does occur. The IUD protects against pregnancy, but when pregnancy occurs it is more likely to be ectopic in location. Overall, women with IUDs have a reduced risk of ectopic pregnancy when compared to women using no form of contraception. Failure rates for IUDs are 0.2–3%. The lower rate approximates those associated with female sterilization and is encountered with the use of new levo-norgestrel-releasing products. Depending on the product, IUDs can remain safely in place for 1–10 years, making them a user-friendly form of contraception.

Hormonal contraception

Combination oral contraceptive pills (OCPs) are the most widely used form of hormonal contraception. They include a synthetic oestrogen (ethinyl oestradiol or mestranol) combined with a variety of synthetic progestins taken orally for 21 consecutive days of every 28. The progestin component of combination OCPs varies in its activity on progesterone receptors, androgen receptors and mineralocorticoid receptors. The oestrogen and progestin dosages in combination OCPs may be constant over the 21 days or may be sequentially modulated (phased or triphasic pills). Combination OCPs prevent pregnancy by multiple mechanisms, including inhibition of ovulation, thickening of cervical mucus to prevent sperm transport and alteration of the uterine lining to block implantation.

OCPs appear to have some health benefits beyond pregnancy prevention, including decreased risks for pelvic inflammatory diseases (PID), benign breast disease, anaemia and endometrial and ovarian cancer. They are not totally risk free, however, and are associated with increased risk of thromboembolic disease, non-thrombotic stroke and gallbladder disease. Women over 35 who smoke should not use OCPs. Failure rates are 0.5–2%. To be effective, OCPs must be taken in the correct order on a daily basis.

Combinations of oestrogen and progestin are now available for contraception in non-oral formulations. These include transdermal patches, injections and vaginal rings. Although still new, all may have efficacy similar to combination OCPs, but with reduced metabolic side-effect profiles (e.g. reduced thromboembolic complications).

Progestin-only contraceptives can be administered orally or parenterally. Both work by thickening cervical mucus and altering the endometrial lining of the uterus, so preventing sperm from reaching the site of fertilization and any fertilized eggs from implanting. In some women, progestin alone will also prevent ovulation. The oral form of the progestin-only contraceptive is known as the 'mini-pill', and is useful in women with contraindications to oestrogen such as breastfeeding. The mini-pill has a failure rate of 1–3%, slightly higher than that of the combination pill, and requires exquisite timing of administration to maximize efficacy.

Depo-Provera is the injectable form of contraceptive progestin. It is given as an intramuscular injection every 90 days. Norplant is a system of six soft capsules of progestin that are implanted under the skin. They release progestin slowly and may be left in place for 5 years. Norplant is currently unavailable in the USA, but continues to be used worldwide. Similar implantable progestin-releasing products are in development. The advantage of the parenteral forms of hormonal contraception is that, once in place, they require no effort by the user. The disadvantage is that they are not readily reversible. In cases of serious side-effects or a desire for pregnancy, one must wait for Depo-Provera to clear the system or have an implantable device surgically removed. The failure rate for Depo-Provera is 1%, and for Norplant 0.2–1.6%.

Emergency hormonal contraception ('morning-after pill') can be effective in preventing pregnancy if taken within 72 h of unprotected intercourse or a contraceptive failure. It uses the same hormones, but in higher doses, and the same mechanisms for preventing pregnancy, as found in combination OCPs. Emergency contraception involving combinations of oestrogen and progestin is associated with more gastric disturbances than that using progestin alone.

Sterilization

Sterilization of both men and women are surgical methods of permanent contraception. Sterilization prevents the gametes from reaching the point of fertilization. In women, surgical options consist of tubal ligation and hysterectomy. Tubal ligation surgically interrupts the Fallopian tubes and may involve the use of tying, blockade, cautery, partial excision or banding. Interruption of the Fallopian tube prevents egg and sperm interactions. Failure rates for tubal ligation vary with the method used for tubal interruption, but all methods are excellent choices if permanent contraception is desired. Ten-year cumulative failure rates for female sterilization are 0.75–3.5%. If a pregnancy does occur after tubal ligation, it has a 40–50% chance of implantation in an ectopic (tubal) location because of the blockage of the Fallopian tube. Hysterectomies are rarely performed solely for sterilization but do eliminate the possibility of pregnancy.

The sterilization procedure in men is called a **vasectomy**. It involves bilateral interruption of the vas deferens as they leave the testes in the scrotum. Surgical methods for interruption include partial excision, cautery or tying. Vasectomy is typically 100% effective but requires a 3-month waiting period and multiple post-procedure ejaculations to clear the vas deferens of previously produced sperm. Vasectomy is a risk factor for prostate cancer (Chapter 40). Male and female sterilization should be considered permanent. Still, surgical reversal procedures exist for both and success of reversibility depends on the initial method of interruption. In women, tubal reanastomosis is associated with post-procedure pregnancy rates of up to 70–80%. In men, the success rates vary with type of interruption procedure and with time from procedure. If reversal is performed within 3 years of interruption, it is also associated with post-procedure pregnancy rates of up to 70–80%.

Abnormalities of male sexual differentiation and development

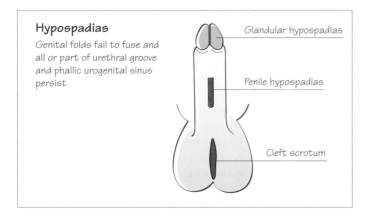

Hypospadias

Genital folds fail to fuse and all or part of urethral groove and phallic urogenital sinus persist

Glandular hypospadias

Penile hypospadias

Cleft scrotum

Cryptorchidism

An undescended testis (cryptorchidism) is the most common genital abnormality seen in male newborns. It occurs in 3% of newborns. Either one or both testes may be involved. Cryptorchidism occurs when the gubernaculum either fails to develop or fails to pull the testes into the scrotum. Androgen activity directs gubernacular development and function, thus gubernacular dysfunction reflects androgen abnormalities. Insufficient androgen activity can result from developmental defects anywhere along the fetal hypothalamic–pituitary–testicular axis. To this point, cryptorchidism can result from any of the following: (i) fetal hypothalamic failure to stimulate gonadotropin secretion in the third trimester (Kallman and Prader–Willi syndromes, anencephaly); (ii) failure of the testes to secrete androgens (gonadal dysgenesis); (iii) failure of testosterone conversion to dihydrotestosterone in target tissues (5α-reductase deficiency); or (iv) absence of functioning androgen receptors (androgen insensitivity syndromes).

Cryptorchid testes may remain in the inguinal canal (70%), the abdomen or retroperitoneum (25%), or other ectopic locations (5%). Testes remaining in the abdomen or inguinal canal will be exposed to comparatively higher temperatures than those of the scrotum and will cease spermatogenesis in response. They are also prone to neoplastic change. Medical therapy for cryptorchidism involves administration of human chorionic gonadotropin (hCG) or androgens. Surgical therapy is called orchiopexy. Some cryptorchid testes are unresponsive to medications or cannot be brought into the scrotum surgically. These testes are usually removed because they cannot be adequately monitored for the development of a neoplasm.

Inguinal hernia is a forme fruste of cryptorchidism. Here, testicular descent occurs, but the inguinal ring does not close completely after descent. Boys who have an inguinal hernia diagnosed before the age of 15 have twice the risk of developing testicular cancer of boys in the general population.

Hypospadias

Another very common congenital abnormality seen in male newborns is hypospadias. In hypospadias, the urethral meatus opens onto the ventral surface of the penile shaft at sites proximal to the normal location. Embryologically, hypospadias results from a failure of complete ventral closure of the urethral groove. The penile urethra depends on the androgen dihydrotestosterone (DHT) to differentiate. Therefore, hypospadias

can result from deficiencies in testosterone (T) production, from inadequate conversion of T to DHT, or from local deficiencies in androgen recognition (insufficient androgen receptor number or function). There is a non-Mendelian genetic predisposition to hypospadias. If one sibling has a hypospadias, the recurrence risk is 12% in that family. If both the father and a brother are affected, the risk for a second son is 25%.

Cryptorchidism is seen in 16% of boys with hypospadias. If both are present, the child may be a pseudohermaphrodite (see below) and chromosomal and hormonal testing should be obtained.

Congenital bilateral absence of the vas deferens

Congenital bilateral absence of the vas deferens (CBAVD) is a rare congenital anomaly found most often in men with cystic fibrosis (CF). It can also occur in the absence of clinically apparent CF. When it does, it is usually associated with mutations in the gene coding for the CF transmembrane receptor (CFTR). The molecular mechanism by which an abnormal transmembrane receptor involved in chloride channels leads either to failure of the vas deferens to differentiate or to its resorption is not known. The presence of CBAVD mandates genetic testing for CF genes.

Pseudohermaphroditism

Individuals possessing testes but in the presence of external and/or internal genitalia with a female phenotype are called male pseudohermaphrodites. Gonadal sex does not match genital phenotype. Male pseudohermaphroditism results from an inappropriate fetal hormonal environment. This can be caused by biochemical defects in androgen activity or by abnormal sex chromosome constitution. Pseudohermaphroditism is a rare disorder, but its multiple aetiologies have offered the opportunity to further understand the role of steroids in human genital development. A list of the known biochemical defects leading to male pseudohermaphroditism includes:

- Androgen insensitivity syndromes.
- 5α-Reductase deficiency.
- Testosterone biosynthesis defects.
- Lipoid congenital adrenal hyperplasia (StAR protein deficiency).
- 3β-Hydroxysteroid dehydrogenase deficiency.
- 17α-Hydroxylase deficiency.
- 17β-Hydroxysteroid dehydrogenase deficiency.
- Impaired androgenization.
- Anti-Müllerian hormone defect.

Androgen insensitivity syndromes

The androgen insensitivity syndromes are a group of X-linked recessive traits that produce a spectrum of incompletely virilized phenotypes. The most severe form, **complete androgen insensitivity (AI)**, was originally known as **testicular feminization**. In complete AI, the intracellular androgen receptor is absent or non-functional. Androgen induction of Wolffian duct development does not occur. Müllerian-inhibiting substance (MIS) is produced by the normally functioning testes and the Müllerian ducts regress. The testes descend to the level of the inguinal ring under the influence of MIS. A short vagina forms from the urogenital sinus. At birth, children with complete AI are typically assigned the female sex because there is no trace of androgen activity and the external genitalia clearly appear female. Complete AI is typically diagnosed after puberty when primary amenorrhoea becomes apparent. Examination of the complete AI individual reveals a blind-ending, short vagina and an absent cervix, uterus and ovaries. Breast development is normal, but axillary and pubic hair is scant or absent. Complete AI accounts for about 10% of all cases of primary amenorrhoea. In contrast to those individuals with a dysgenetic gonad bearing a Y chromosome (see below), those with complete AI have less than a 5% risk of developing a gonadal tumour. Gonadal tumours that do develop in AI patients rarely appear before age 25. Therefore, gonadectomy is postponed until puberty is complete.

The **incomplete androgen insensitivity syndrome (Reifenstein syndrome)** is far less common than the complete and is associated with a broad spectrum of phenotypes. These vary from almost complete failure of internal and external genital virilization to essentially complete phenotypic masculinization. Between these extremes exist patients with mild clitoromegaly and slight labial fusion to those with significant genital ambiguity. Recently, several men have been described whose only indication of AI was infertility resulting from low or absent sperm production. Some fertile males who appear undervirilized probably have a mild form of this disorder.

Incomplete AI results from mutations in the androgen receptor gene. The gene encoding the androgen receptor localizes to the q11–12 region of the X chromosome. Defects can occur in the androgen-binding domain of the receptor, the DNA-binding domain of the receptor or in receptor protein production. Identified abnormalities range from complete loss of receptor function to subtle qualitative changes in the transcription of androgen dependent target genes. There is poor correlation between absolute androgen receptor levels and the degree of masculinization seen in patients with incomplete AI.

5α–Reductase deficiency

The syndrome seen among patients with 5α-reductase deficiency was originally given the name **pseudovaginal perineoscrotal hypospadias (PPH)**. It differs from AI in that masculinization occurs at puberty. At birth, individuals with 5α-reductase deficiency have external genitalia that resemble those of incomplete AI, including hypospadias, varying degrees of failure of the labioscrotal folds to fuse and either a urogenital opening or separate vaginal and urethral openings. The cleft in the scrotum resembles a vagina and most children with 5α-reductase deficiency are raised as girls. In these patients, adrenal steroid production is normal and the karyotype is XY. Measuring blood levels of testosterone and dihydrotestosterone and demonstrating an elevated T:DHT ratio can establish the diagnosis of 5α-reductase deficiency and eliminate the diagnosis of congenital adrenal hyperplasia in an incompletely virilized female newborn (Chapter 27).

Molecular analyses have demonstrated that there are two 5α-reductase genes; mutations in the isoenzyme coded on chromosome 2 (*SRD5A2* gene) are responsible for this form of male pseudohermaphroditism.

Multiple mutations of *SRD5A2* have been identified. The segregation of the same specific defects in unrelated individuals of the same ethnicity suggests common ancestry. Compound heterozygotes are common, suggesting that the gene frequency for *SRD5A2* mutations may be fairly high. Women are not clinically affected by 5α-reductase deficiency.

Congenital adrenal hyperplasia syndromes

A group of enzymatic defects of the steroidogenic pathways cause reproductive and metabolic disorders collectively known as the congenital adrenal hyperplasia (CAH) syndromes. Among these, lipoid congenital adrenal hyperplasia (StAR protein deficiency), 3β-hydroxysteroid dehydrogenase deficiency, 17α-hydroxylase deficiency and 17β-hydroxysteroid dehydrogenase deficiency can cause feminization of fetal external genitalia. All are specific enzymatic defects in the steroidogenic pathway common to the testes and adrenal glands and all involve enzymes occurring early in the steroidogenic pathway between cholesterol and testosterone (Chapters 3 and 29). CAH syndromes that cause masculinization in female fetuses are much more common and result from enzymatic defects more distal in the steroidogenic pathways.

Gender assignment

Gender assignment in male infants with pseudohermaphroditism requires knowledge of the specific defect. Most are raised as females. Individuals with complete AI (testicular feminization) are raised as females because they unambiguously appear as females at birth. In addition, because they lack functional androgen receptors, AI patients will never be virilized. Males whose incomplete AI presents with ambiguous genitalia are also usually raised as females because predictable feminization with gynaecomastia will occur at puberty. Males with 5α-reductase deficiency have been successfully raised as either females or males. In fact, in cultures with a high frequency of the disorder, children have been raised as females in childhood and males after puberty. Patients with 5α-reductase deficiency who are assigned as females and wish to retain their female gender will need to be gonadectomized to avoid deepening of their voices and a male pattern of muscle development that will occur at puberty. Both will occur in response to pubertal testosterone, a substance to which they can respond. Oestrogen and progesterone therapy can be used to produce female secondary sexual development. Patients with 5α-reductase deficiency who are assigned to the male gender require repair of their hypospadias and cryptorchidism. At puberty, spermatogenesis and masculine sexual maturation will occur under the influence of testosterone.

True gonadal dysgenesis is relatively rare in individuals with an XY karyotype. Bilateral dysgenesis of the testes (**Swyer syndrome**) results in normal, but infantile female external and internal genital development and lack of secondary sexual development at puberty. Fibrous bands appear in place of the testes. Gonadectomy is necessary to prevent the 20–30% risk of tumour formation. Oestrogen and progesterone therapy support female secondary sexual development at puberty.

The androgen insensitivity syndromes

	Complete	Reifenstein	Infertile	5α-Reductase
Inheritance	X-linked recessive	X-linked recessive	X-linked recessive	Autosomal recessive
Spermatogenesis	Absent	Absent	Decreased	Decreased
Müllerian structures	Absent	Absent	Absent	Absent
Wolffian structures	Absent	Male	Male	Male
External genitalia	Female	Male/hypospadias	Male	Female
Breasts (puberty)	Female	Female/gynaecomastia	Gynaecomastia	Male

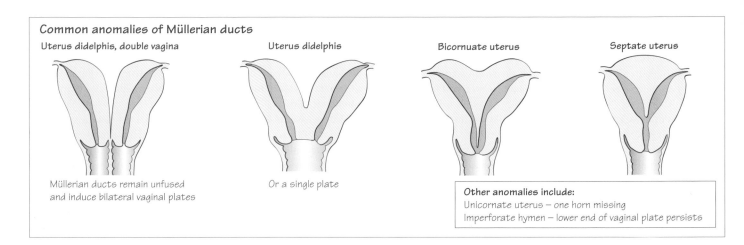

Common anomalies of Müllerian ducts

Uterus didelphis, double vagina

Müllerian ducts remain unfused
and induce bilateral vaginal plates

Uterus didelphis

Or a single plate

Bicornuate uterus

Septate uterus

Other anomalies include:
Unicornate uterus – one horn missing
Imperforate hymen – lower end of vaginal plate persists

Structural anomalies

Structural anomalies of the uterus, cervix and vagina are the most common abnormalities of sexual differentiation seen in women. They arise from embryological abnormalities of Müllerian system development (Chapters 6 and 7). The most severe form involves complete absence of the reproductive tract, including the vagina, uterus and Fallopian tubes. Such agenesis of the Müllerian system is known as Mayer–Rokitansky–Kuster–Hauser syndrome, and is the second most common cause of primary amenorrhoea (see Chapter 30).

The remainder of the anomalies result from failure of the Müllerian system to fuse in the midline or to remodel in the midline after fusion to form a single uterine cavity. The most dramatic form of fusion anomalies occurs when the Müllerian ducts fail to fuse along their entire length, resulting in the formation of two vaginas, two cervices and two separate uterine horns (double uterus or *uterus didelphis*). More commonly, only the upper portion of the uterus fails to fuse. The uterine body may then remain separated as two horns (bicornuate uterus or *uterus bicornus*) or, in milder cases, a dimple may be noted in the contour of the uterine fundus (arcuate uterus). Occasionally, only one side of the Müllerian system will develop, resulting in a hemi-uterus and a single Fallopian tube (unicornuate uterus or *uterus unicornus*).

Failure to resorb the midline of the Müllerian ducts after fusion typically results in a uterine septum. A septum may be complete, running from the cervix to the fundus, or incomplete, involving only the uterine fundus (subseptate uterus). Occasionally the vagina canalizes improperly and a vaginal septum will occur. This can occur in isolation or in conjunction with a uterine anomaly. Vaginal septa can be either longitudinal or horizontal. The longitudinal septum is reminiscent of those uterine anomalies resulting from failure of the Müllerian midline to resorb. Horizontal vaginal septa are thought to represent a failure of the vaginal plate to resorb at the site where it fuses with the Müllerian ducts.

Many women with structural anomalies of the reproductive tract are asymptomatic and never diagnosed. Others with Müllerian tract abnormalities may present with primary amenorrhoea, recurrent miscarriages, preterm delivery and breech presentation at term. **Because the mesonephros is closely involved in directing the development of the internal genitalia, the finding of a uterine anomaly should prompt an evaluation of the urinary system for an accompanying anomaly.**

Exposure to diethylstilbestrol

In utero exposure to diethylstilbestrol (DES) occurred in individuals born between 1940 and 1972 whose mothers were given the synthetic oestrogen in the hope of preventing a miscarriage. DES was subsequently shown to cause congenital abnormalities in women and, to a lesser degree, in men. The most frequently seen abnormalities in women are abnormally shaped cervices. These cervices have been described as coxcomb, hooded or hypoplastic. The uterine musculature may also be abnormally formed in DES-exposed women such that the cavity assumes a T-shape on hysterosalpingography. DES appears to cause these abnormalities via inappropriate activation of oestrogen-dependent genes involved in differentiating the cervix and upper third of the vagina from the lower vagina. This results not only in the structurally abnormal cervices and uteri, but also in persistence of cervical glandular epithelium in the vagina (**vaginal adenosis**). *In utero* DES exposure is associated with an increased risk of reproductive failure, including infertility (likely from failed implantation), recurrent pregnancy loss and preterm delivery. DES daughters are also at increased risk for malignancies arising in sites of vaginal adenosis. This is thought to result from exposure of the ectopic cervical glandular-type epithelia in the vagina to neoplastic inducers not usually accessible to the upper reproductive tract.

Occasionally, clinicians will observe cervical and uterine abnormalities that look exactly like those caused by *in utero* DES exposure in women never exposed to DES.

Congenital adrenal hyperplasia

Ambiguous genitalia in a newborn infant are most commonly caused by congenital adrenal hyperplasia (CAH). This diagnosis accounts for 40–50% of all cases of ambiguous genitalia. Depending on the degree of the defect and the particular steroidogenic enzyme that is dysfunctional, neonatal effects can be variable. Affected female infants may have a common urogenital sinus containing the vagina and urethra, which opens at the base of an enlarged phallus resembling a penis. The labia majora may be hypertrophied or fused and thus resemble an empty scrotum. Some female infants will appear like a male with hypospadias and cryptorchidism. Others will only exhibit mild to moderate clitoromegaly. Some of these infants will have accompanying hypertension (5%) or life-threatening salt wasting (30%) and this will aid in making the diagnosis soon after birth. Those carrying the most common defect, moderate 21β-hydroxylase deficiency, will have no other identifying characteristics. **The finding of a normal female karyotype in a newborn assigned to the male gender in the delivery room requires an evaluation for CAH.**

The primary defect in all types of CAH is the absence of one of the enzymes necessary for steroidogenesis. The most common forms involve the enzymes that convert androgens to the adrenal steroids (see table below). In the absence of one of these enzymes, no steroidal endproduct will be produced by the adrenal gland to feed back on the hypothalamic–pituitary axis and regulate adrenocorticotropic hormone (ACTH) secretion. Excess ACTH will continue to stimulate the adrenals to produce more of the steroid products prior to the enzymatic block. These products are then shunted toward androgen-forming pathways. Adrenal hyperplasia with excess androgen production will result. This is of little consequence in the male fetus but will result in masculinization of the androgen-sensitive external genitalia in a female fetus. Because the female fetus has neither testes nor Müllerian-inhibiting substance (MIS), females affected by CAH will have uteri and vaginas. The degree of hypertrophy and fusion of the external genitalia in CAH females will depend on the quantity of androgen involved and on the developmental timing of androgen exposure. Masculinized infants with ovaries and a 46XX karyotype are called female pseudohermaphrodites.

Therapy for **female infants masculinized as a result of CAH** includes glucocorticoid administration to suppress adrenal androgen secretion and genital reconstructive surgery. Infants who also have a defect in aldosterone synthesis will also require mineralocorticoid replacement.

Virilization of female infants by maternal or exogenous androgen exposure occurs only when those androgens are unable to be converted to oestrogens by placental aromatase. Therefore, infants born to mothers with CAH are not at risk unless the child has inherited the genetic defect from both parents and also carries the enzymatic deficiency. Infants born to mothers with an androgen-producing tumour may be virilized if the particular androgen produced cannot be aromatized (e.g. dihydrotestosterone, DHT) or it quantitatively exceeds the high aromatization capacity of the placenta. Maternal administration of synthetic progestins with androgenic activity has also been associated with virilization of the female neonate; use of synthetic progesterones is contraindicated in pregnant women. Female virilization that has resulted from *in utero* steroid exposure but has no accompanying risk for postnatal exposure can be treated with reconstructive surgery alone.

Turner syndrome

Women with Turner syndrome are often identified when the physical characteristics of short stature, webbed neck, shield chest and increased carrying angle accompany primary amenorrhoea. The fundamental defect in Turner syndrome patients is the absence of a second sex chromosome, i.e. a 45X karyotype. In the absence of a functional second sex chromosome, the germ cells in the gonad do not survive past the embryonic period and a normal ovary or testis does not develop. Gonadal steroid synthesis and secretion do not occur during embryogenesis or at puberty. Systems other than reproduction are affected by Turner syndrome. Women with the disorder have an increased incidence of renal anomalies, autoimmune diseases and cardiac anomalies, particularly coarctation of the aorta and aortic aneurysms. Turner syndrome is the most common of a group of disorders known as **gonadal dysgenesis**.

Most individuals with gonadal dysgenesis have a female phenotype at birth. If the entirety of the second sex chromosome is missing, both the external and internal genitalia will be female. After puberty, these female structures will remain infantile because of the lack of ovarian oestrogens from the non-functional gonad. If any remnant of a second sex chromosome is present in an individual with gonadal dysgenesis, the phenotype will depend on the specific genes retained. For instance, if the SRY locus is present and translocated onto another chromosome, signals to begin testicular differentiation will occur. MIS will be produced and the Müllerian duct system will regress. Despite MIS production, these individuals will have a rudimentary testis and lack androgen production. They will be born with female external genitalia, but lack a vagina and other female internal reproductive structures. Primordial Wolffian ducts may be identified at laparotomy along with ovotestes. These rare individuals are true hermaphrodites.

Sex chromosome **mosaicism** (multiple cell lines of different sex chromosomal composition) is not uncommon in Turner syndrome. Individuals carrying any portion of the Y chromosome, including SRY alone, may have a testicular component to their dysgenetic gonad. These patients are at risk for gonadal malignancies and may have functional testicular tissue that causes virilization at puberty. Therefore it is important to confirm any suspected diagnosis of Turner syndrome using karyotype analysis. Some experts recommend using a DNA probe against SRY as well. Individuals who possess a cell line containing a Y chromosome or who carry SRY should undergo bilateral gonadectomy prior to puberty to eliminate the possibility of virilization or cancer.

If sex chromosome mosaicism involves a second X chromosome, functional ovarian tissue may exist within the gonad. Women with such mosaicism may experience normal female puberty and even retain fertility for a brief period of time. Early menopause invariably occurs because the abnormal chromosomal constitution causes development of only a limited number of functional ovarian follicles. A woman with complete Turner syndrome or XX mosaicism can carry a pregnancy conceived through *in vitro* fertilization using donated oocytes. Her infantile uterus will require extensive hormonal priming.

'Virilizing' forms of congenital adrenal hyperplasia

Enzyme deficiency	Clinical appearance	Cortisol	Aldosterone	Androgens
21β-Hydroxylase—severe	Salt-wasting, virilized	−	−	++
21β-Hydroxylase—moderate	Virilized	Normal	+	++
21β-Hydroxylase—mild	Adult polycystic ovaries	Normal	+/−	+
11β-Hydroxylase	Hypertensive, virilized	−	−	++
17α-Hydroxylase	Hypertensive	−	+/−	−

Precocious puberty

Sexual precocity is defined as the appearance of secondary sexual characteristics before the age of 8 years in girls and before the age of 9 years in boys. Recent data suggest that these ages are less than two standard deviations from the mean. Still, the ramifications of misdiagnosis are great and, at present, breast or pubic hair development before age 8 or menarche before age 10 warrants an evaluation in girls. Testicular enlargement or pubic hair development before age 9 in boys warrants similar investigation. While the appearance of all secondary sex characteristics results from increased sex steroid production, the underlying aetiology of elevated sex hormone production and activity may be increased gonadotropin secretion or intrinsic disease of the adrenal, ovary or testis. **Complete or true sexual precocity** is used to describe precocious puberty resulting from elevated pituitary gonadotropins. **Incomplete or peripheral sexual precocity** refers to precocious puberty resulting from primary diseases of the gonads or adrenals. Early sexual development that is consistent with the genetic and gonadal sex of the individual is **isosexual precocity**. **Heterosexual** or **contrasexual precocity** indicates precocious puberty associated with feminization of a male or virilization of a female.

Although more than half the cases of isosexual precocious puberty simply represent the early end of the normal developmental spectrum, all children with sexual precocity should be evaluated. There are several reasons for this recommendation. First, some children may be suffering from a serious disorder associated with precocious puberty. Second, regardless of the aetiology, sexual development that occurs before age 6–7 years can be associated with short stature in adulthood if left untreated. Finally, **sexual precocity is not accompanied by advanced psychosexual maturation**. To this point, young girls with precocious puberty appear to be at significant risk for sexual abuse. Ovulation and conception are possible and pregnancies in girls as young as 5 years of age have occurred as the result of such abuse. Appropriate therapy and support are necessary to prevent the potential long-term consequences of sexual precocity.

True or complete precocious puberty

True sexual precocity results from early maturation of the hypothalamic–pituitary–gonadal (H-P-G) axis. Measurements of serum gonadotropins and sex steroid concentrations will be in the normal postpubertal range. Gonadotropin pulsatility will have characteristics and feedback regulation similar to those found in the adult. The physical characteristics of puberty appear prematurely, but in the proper chronological order. One half of cases of true sexual precocity arise from premature activation of the H-P-G axis.

The remaining cases of complete isosexual precocity are caused by central nervous system (CNS) lesions. These lesions include neoplasms, trauma, hydrocephalus, postinfectious encephalitis, congenital brain defects, tuberous sclerosis and neurofibromatosis type I. Most lesions are located in, or near, the posterior hypothalamus. The most commonly identified neoplasms are astrocytomas, ependymomas and craniopharyngiomas. Hamartomas of the tuber cinereum account for one in six cases of isosexual precocious puberty in girls and half of the cases in boys. Hamartomas are congenital malformations that contain fibre bundles, glial cells and gonadotropin-releasing hormone (GnRH)-secreting neurons.

Although it is a rare cause of precocious puberty, girls with severe primary hypothyroidism can develop hyperprolactinaemia, associated galactorrhea and true precocious puberty. These girls have a primary defect in their thyroid gland and very high thyroid-stimulating hormone (TSH) levels in response to low thyroid hormone secretion. They also have elevated circulating gonadotropins. The development of precocious puberty in girls with primary hypothyroidism may be the direct result of gonadotropin stimulation of the ovary or may result from cross-activation of the follicle-stimulating hormone (FSH) receptor by the pathologically high TSH. In the face of low thyroid hormone secretion, hypothalamic thyrotropin-releasing hormone (TRH) production rises. TRH is a potent stimulator of prolactin secretion by pituitary lactotrophs (Chapter 1); hyperprolactinaemia and galactorrhoea result.

Occasionally, the development of true sexual precocity will follow the correction of a long-standing virilizing condition in girls. This may occur with treatment of congenital adrenal hyperplasia. Correction of excess androgen production releases the hypothalamus from androgen-associated negative feedback. This permits GnRH secretion and gonadotropin stimulation of the ovary. The timing of this stimulation may be inappropriate and, in a young girl, lead to complete precocious isosexual development.

Treatment of true precocious puberty involves recognition and correction of underlying CNS lesions if aetiological. Additional therapy may be required, including suppression of the H-P-G axis with a GnRH agonist or antagonist. GnRH agonists are long-acting analogues of GnRH that occupy its receptors for extended periods of time. Prolonged receptor occupation removes the GnRH pulsatility necessary for gonadotropin release from the pituitary. GnRH antagonists occupy and block GnRH receptors and cause immediate cessation of GnRH pulsatility. Both can be effective in protecting adult height and avoiding many psychosexual issues surrounding untreated precocious puberty.

Incomplete isosexual precocity

Incomplete isosexual precocity is caused by ovarian or adrenal secretion of oestrogen in girls and testicular or adrenal secretion of androgen in boys.

In girls, the most common cause of GnRH-independent precocious puberty is the presence of functionally autonomous ovarian cysts. Small (<1 cm) follicles occur frequently in the prepubertal ovary but they rarely secrete significant amounts of oestrogen. However, autonomous secretion of oestradiol by the granulosa cells contained in the cyst wall can occur in larger cysts, and serum oestradiol concentrations appear to correlate directly with cyst size. Progestin therapy can reduce the size of these cysts and prevent their recurrence.

Solid stromal cell tumours of the ovary are a rare cause of GnRH-independent precocious puberty in girls. When compared to functional cysts of the ovary, juvenile granulosa or theca cell tumours secrete very large amount of oestrogen, often resulting in the rapid development of sexual characteristics.

Two inherited syndromes, Peutz–Jeghers and McCune–Albright, are associated with isosexual precocious puberty. Peutz–Jeghers syndrome is defined by the appearance of mucocutaneous pigmentation and gastrointestinal polyposis, but may also include gonadal sex cord tumours. McCune–Albright syndrome is characterized by hyperpigmented café-au-lait spots on the skin, progressive polyostotic fibrous dysplasia of the bones, and GnRH-independent sexual precocity. Hyperplasia or adenomas of multiple endocrine glands may also occur. McCune–Albright syndrome is caused by activating mutations in a signal transduction protein linked to many of the peptide hormone receptors, the G-protein subunit, $G_s\alpha$. These proteins are present in many cells and therefore many tissues can be affected; distribution may be patchy and unpredictable because mutations occur in postzygotic somatic cells. In girls with McCune–Albright syndrome and ovarian involvement, sexual precocity occurs because of oestrogen secretion from luteinized follicular cysts and treatment involves interruption of oestrogen production. CNS involvement is unlikely and patients with McCune–Albright syndrome can progress normally through GnRH-dependent puberty.

Incomplete isosexual precocious puberty is rare in boys. It is always caused by excess androgen exposure. Adrenal sources of androgen exposure include congenital adrenal hyperplasia and adrenal adenomas or cancers. Most virilizing adrenal tumours in children secrete excess amounts of dehydroepiandrosterone sulfate (DHEA-S). The DHEA-S, in turn, is converted to more potent androgens (Chapter 3). Testicular sources of androgen excess include Leydig cell tumours. These rare tumours of the testis produce testosterone.

Iatrogenic sexual precocity

Breast development has been reported in girls and boys after exposure to exogenous oestrogens found in tonics, lotions, creams and oestrogen-contaminated meat. Virilization of boys and girls has been associated with exposure to androgenic steroid preparations.

Virilizing precocious puberty in girls

Most girls with contrasexual precocious puberty will develop pubic hair or hirsutism. The most common cause is congenital adrenal hyperplasia. CAH is associated with multiple defects in the steroid synthetic pathway. Mild alterations in adrenal 21-hydroxylase are present in 0.1–1.0% of the population. These alterations may not manifest themselves as early as those of classical CAH; mild deficiencies are associated with late virilization, premature adrenarche, polycystic ovarian disease or postpubertal oligoamenorrhoea. The diagnosis of this disorder rests on the presence of mild baseline elevations in 17-hydroxyprogesterone, the steroid precursor metabolized by 21-hydroxylase. Some patients with the disorder will be discovered only after provocative testing, characterized by the exaggerated release of 17-hydroxyprogesterone to adrenocorticotropic hormone (ACTH) stimulation. Deficiencies in 11β-hydroxylase deficiency or 3β-hydroxysteroid dehydrogenase can cause virilizing precocious puberty in girls, but occur rarely.

Virilizing adrenal tumours that occur in young girls are very aggressive and usually fatal if malignant. Ovarian Leydig cell and Sertoli cell tumours are the most common virilizing neoplasms in women. They are a rare cause of virilizing precocious puberty.

Feminizing precocious puberty in boys

Contrasexual precocity is much less common in boys than in girls. Boys with feminizing precocious puberty will exhibit gynaecomastia and accelerated linear bone growth. The presence of prepubertal-size testes on examination strongly suggests an adrenal or testicular source for the oestrogen. One rare cause of prepubertal feminization is extraglandular aromatization of androstenedione. Gynaecomastia has occasionally been seen with congenital adrenal hyperplasia in boys. Feminizing testicular tumours have been reported in boys with Peutz–Jeghers syndrome.

Classification of precocious puberty

Complete isosexual precocity (true precocious puberty—gonadotropin dependent)
Idiopathic
CNS lesions
  Hamartomas
  Craniopharyngioma
Primary hypothyroidism
Following treatment for virilizing disorders in girls

Incomplete isosexual precocity (GnRH independent)
Oestrogen-secreting neoplasms of ovary or adrenal in girls
Ovarian cysts
Androgen-secreting neoplasms of testis or adrenal in boys
McCune–Albright syndrome
Peutz–Jeghers syndrome

Iatrogenic sexual precocity

Contrasexual precocity
Virilization in females
  Congenital adrenal hyperplasia
  21-Hydroxylase deficiency
  11β-Hydroxylase deficiency
  3β-Hydroxysteroid dehydrogenase deficiency
  Androgen-secreting ovarian or adrenal neoplasms
Feminization in males
  Oestrogen-secreting adrenal neoplasms

Differential diagnosis of isosexual precocious puberty

	Serum gonadotropin concentration	LH response to GnRH	Serum sex steroid concentrations	Gonadal size	Miscellaneous
True precocious puberty (premature activation of hypothalamic GnRH pulse generator)	Prominent LH pulses	Pubertal LH response	Pubertal	Normal pubertal	MRI scan to rule out CNS abnormality, bone scan to exclude McCune–Albright syndrome
Incomplete sexual precocity (GnRH independent) Girls					
Follicular cysts	Low	Suppressed	Varies	Ovarian enlargement	Exclude McCune–Albright syndrome
Granulosa cell tumour	Low	Suppressed	Very high oestradiol	Ovarian enlargement	Tumour may be palpable
Feminizing adrenal tumour	Low	Suppressed	High oestradiol and DHEA-S	Prepubertal ovaries	Unilateral adrenal mass
Boys Congenital adrenal hyperplasia	Low	Suppressed	High 17-hydroxyprogesterone	Prepubertal testes	
Virilizing adrenal tumours	Low	Suppressed	High DHEA-S	Prepubertal	Unilateral adrenal mass
Leydig/Sertoli cell tumour	Low	Suppressed	High testosterone	Testicular mass	

LH, luteinizing hormone; MRI, magnetic resonance imaging.

Delayed or absent puberty

Delayed puberty is defined as the absence of secondary sexual characteristics at age 13 in girls and 16 in boys (Chapters 12 and 13). It may result from: (i) a non-pathological **constitutional delay** accompanying a growth delay; (ii) disorders of the hypothalamus or pituitary gland that result in inadequate gonadotropin secretion (**hypogonadotropic hypogonadism**); and (iii) disorders of the gonads that prevent adequate sex steroid secretion (**hypergonadotropic hypogonadism**). In girls, secondary sexual characteristics may develop without progression to menarche. This form of pubertal dysfunction and other causes of primary amenorrhoea are discussed in Chapter 30.

It is important to diagnose and treat delayed or absent puberty because: (i) serious underlying conditions may be present; (ii) abnormal persistence of a child-like phenotype has profound social implications for the teenager and young adult; (iii) prolonged absence of gonadal steroid exposure leads to osteopenia, a failure of normal bone formation. Osteopenia is associated with an increased risk of fractures in weight-bearing bones such as vertebrae, hips and long bones. Treatment of delayed or absent puberty aims to correct underlying disorders. Hormone replacement with oestrogen/progesterone or testosterone is often required if hypogonadism is prolonged or age-appropriate sex steroid secretion patterns cannot be restored.

Constitutional pubertal delay

Pathological causes of delayed puberty must be excluded before the diagnosis of constitutional pubertal delay can be considered. Constitutional pubertal delay is characterized by linear growth velocities and gonadotropin-releasing hormone (GnRH) secretory patterns that are appropriate for the individual's bone age. In girls, it has been observed that puberty begins at a bone age of 12 years. Therefore, a 13-year-old girl who has a bone age of 11 and has not developed secondary sexual characteristics may have constitutional delay.

Hypogonadotropic hypogonadism

This is characterized by **deficiencies in pulsatile GnRH, follicle-stimulating hormone (FSH) or luteinizing hormone (LH) secretion** that result in sexual infantilism. GnRH deficiencies arise via three general mechanisms: genetic defects of the hypothalamus, developmental defects of the hypothalamus and destructive lesions involving the hypothalamus or pituitary stalk.

The best characterized and most common of the genetic defects producing hypogonadotropic hypogonadism is **Kallman syndrome**, which is typified by GnRH deficiency associated with hyposmia and hypoplasia of the olfactory lobes of the brain. It is inherited either as an X-linked recessive trait or as an autosomal dominant trait with variable penetrance. Kallman syndrome is much more common in boys than in girls. Half of Kallman syndrome patients have mutations in the *KAL* gene on chromosome Xp22.3. This gene encodes an extracellular matrix protein that regulates axonal pathfinding and cellular adhesion. Deficiencies in the amounts, or function, of this protein explain the cluster of abnormalities associated with Kallman syndrome: fetal GnRH neurosecretory neurons fail to migrate normally from the olfactory placode to the medial basal hypothalamus, resulting in inappropriate olfactory bulb development, anosmia and GnRH deficiencies.

Less common developmental defects have been associated with delayed or absent puberty due to hypogonadotropic hypogonadism.

These also affect midline central nervous system (CNS) development. Some have been described in association with visual abnormalities that result from developmental abnormalities in the optic tracts. GnRH deficiencies are often associated with other hypothalamic–pituitary functional abnormalities. As a result, delayed puberty is typically accompanied by short stature [growth hormone (GH) deficiency]. This can make differentiation from constitutional delay challenging. A familial form of isolated gonadotropin deficiency has also been described. Unlike most other forms of hypogonadotropic hypogonadism in which GH is also deficient, patients with familial isolated gonadotropin deficiency have normal height for bone age.

CNS tumours result in delayed puberty more often than precocious puberty. Most neoplasms that interfere with pubertal development are extrasellar and inhibit the production, or delivery, of the pituitary trophic hormones to the pituitary gland. Deficiencies in multiple pituitary hormones are common. Of these tumours, craniopharyngiomas are the most common cause of delayed or absent puberty. They originate from cells within the developmental anlagen of the anterior pituitary–Rathke's pouch, and are almost always located in or near the hypothalamus or pituitary. Many pituitary tumours that are common in adults are notably rare in prepubertal children. One, the prolactin-secreting adenomas, may occur among teenagers. Girls with prolactin-secreting pituitary adenomas may present to their medical provider with complaints of primary amenorrhoea in the presence of secondary sexual characteristics. Neurofibromas of the CNS that develop as part of von Recklinghausen syndrome (neurofibromatosis) and germ-cell tumours can also be associated with sexual infantilism.

Functional gonadotropin deficiencies can arise from malnutrition, psychiatric disorders, and from a large array of chronic diseases. Girls seem more sensitive than boys to the effects of malnutrition. In girls, a reduction to less than 80% of ideal body weight can be associated with delayed or arrested puberty. By contrast, starvation of famine proportions is necessary to interfere with male puberty.

Anorexia nervosa is a serious psychiatric disorder characterized by a distorted body image, an obsessive fear of obesity and associated food avoidance. It can cause severe, and sometimes fatal, weight loss. While not restricted by age or gender, anorexia nervosa is far more common in girls than in boys and most often begins during adolescence. It is associated with delayed puberty, and can be accompanied by primary or secondary amenorrhoea, depending on the age at onset. The hypogonadotropic hypogonadism of anorexia nervosa is related only in part to the weight loss associated with the disorder. In fact, in postpubertal girls, secondary amenorrhoea may precede severe weight loss. Affected individuals will have a reversion of LH secretion to a prepubertal circadian rhythm. Recovery of normal weight will correct many of the coexisting endocrine and metabolic abnormalities, including: low cortisol and triiodothyronine, increased GH and decreased IGF-I and a blunted pituitary response to trophic hormones. The amenorrhoea accompanying anorexia nervosa may persist long after otherwise adequate weight gain. Bulimia nervosa, a variant of anorexia nervosa associated with food gorging, induced vomiting and laxative abuse, produces amenorrhoea unassociated with weight loss. This suggests the amenorrhoea of anorexia and bulimia nervosa may have a primary hypothalamic origin.

Intense exercise and athletic training may delay or arrest puberty due to inhibition of GnRH secretion. Again, this is more common in girls than in boys. Distance runners, gymnasts and dancers are at highest risk. Interruption of the intense training by injury advances puberty before weight gain occurs, suggesting a direct effect of the physical activity on GnRH secretion. Female athletes with normal body weight, but less body fat than non-athletic girls (e.g. swimmers and ice skaters) are also at risk for hypogonadotropic hypogonadism and delayed puberty.

Hypergonadotropic hypogonadism

Gonadal dysgenesis is the most common cause of hypergonadotropic hypogonadism. Primary gonadal failure results in decreased or absent gonadal steroid secretion. Lack of adequate circulating oestrogen or androgen diminishes negative feedback actions of the hypothalamus on pituitary gland and results in elevated FSH and LH secretion.

Klinefelter syndrome is the most common cause of gonadal dysgenesis, occurring in 1 in 500–1000 of all phenotypic boys. Typical features of the Klinefelter phenotype are a eunuch-like body habitus, gynaecomastia and small testes. The testes of most Klinefelter patients have a distinctly limited capacity to secrete testosterone. The Leydig cells in the testis do not respond normally to LH or FSH stimulation; plasma testosterone levels range from 10% of normal in severely eunuchoid boys to about 50% of normal in those less severely affected. Oestrogen production is also proportionally elevated compared to the amount of testosterone produced, and gynaecomastia is a frequent clinical finding. Boys with Klinefelter syndrome who have circulating testosterone levels in the low normal range will demonstrate puberty and normal height. Those with extremely low circulating testosterone levels will be very tall because of the failure of the epiphyses to close in a timely fashion. Most men with Klinefelter syndrome have normal adrenal androgen production; most will have pubic hair, regardless of circulating testosterone levels.

Boys with Klinefelter syndrome have a progressive loss of spermatogenic activity in the testes after puberty. In normal pubertal boys, about 80% of the seminiferous tubules will contain spermatogonia. In boys with Klinefelter syndrome, only 20% of tubules will contain germ cells. This percentage will decline as the tubules progressively sclerose. Adult men with Klinefelter syndrome are infertile. Most will require androgen replacement therapy to obtain or maintain an adult male phenotype.

Ninety per cent of men with Klinefelter syndrome have a **47XXY karyotype**. The other 10% will display an array of extra X chromosome states. Some will have a 46XX karyotype with translocation of the male sex-determining region (SRY) onto the X chromosome (Chapter 6). Still others will carry additional X chromosomal material as a mosaicism. Klinefelter mosaics account for the largest proportion of affected men who retain partial testicular function. Fertile 46XY mosaics have been reported.

Turner syndrome is the second most common form of gonadal dysgenesis, occurring in about 1/5000 liveborn girls. Typical features of the Turner phenotype include short stature, short webbed neck, micrognathia, broad shield-like chest, anomalies of the left side of the heart (coarctation of the aorta, aortic stenosis, bicuspid aortic valve and dissecting aortic aneurysms) and renal and gastrointestinal anomalies. The ovaries of women with Turner syndrome are typically replaced by connective tissue and are called streak gonads. True streak gonads contain no germ cells and cannot produce reproductive steroids. The uterus and Fallopian tubes are present in women with Turner syndrome, but they typically remain infantile due to lack of oestrogen stimulation. External genitalia and gender orientation are female.

The karyotype of a woman with Turner syndrome is typically **45X**. Like Klinefelter syndrome, structural abnormalities of the X chromosome and mosaicism are also common. Mosaicism and structural abnormalities account for the varied phenotypes reported with the syndrome, which range from that described above to both normal males and females. Of conceptuses with the 45X karyotype, 99% spontaneously abort (miscarry). This supports the systemic nature of the abnormalities seen with complete absence of the second sex chromosome and suggests that most surviving Turner syndrome women are undiagnosed mosaics.

Patients with Turner syndrome are usually smaller than average at birth. They grow normally for the first few years after infancy and then begin to slow. Most fail to demonstrate a pubertal growth spurt. This characteristic growth defect appears to be related to the single copy of a gene on the X chromosome known as *PHOG* or *SHOX*. *PHOG* is a transcription factor expressed in osteoblasts.

Some patients with Turner syndrome will have complex karyotypes with mosaicism involving the Y chromosome. The presence of all or part of the Y chromosome may result in phenotypes with the classic Turner phenotype described above but ambiguous genitalia or normal male external genitalia. Such patients may have gonadal structures ranging from a streak gonad to a functioning testis. Individuals with a Y cell line or abnormalities involving the Y chromosome are at an increased risk for neoplastic transformation in their gonads. Gonadectomy should be performed at the time of diagnosis.

Genetic disorders of steroidogenesis can cause delayed puberty. They are a large group of rare disorders that cause hypergonadotropic hypogonadism. Because most of these autosomal recessive disorders also affect adrenal steroid biosynthesis, they are more commonly known as the **congenital adrenal hyperplasia (CAH) syndromes**. The CAH syndromes associated with delayed puberty are listed in the table below. All these enzyme defects occur in the steroidogenic pathway between cholesterol and testosterone.

Classification of delayed or absent puberty

Constitutional delay in growth and puberty

Hypogonadotropic hypogonadism
CNS disorders
    Congenital malformations
    Destructive lesions
Tumours
Radiation therapy
Kallman syndrome (isolated gonadotropin deficiency)
Multiple pituitary hormone deficiencies
Miscellaneous disorders
Prader–Willi syndrome
Functional gonadotropin deficiency
    Chronic systemic disease and malnutrition
    Hypothyroidism
    Cushing disease
    Diabetes mellitus
    Hyperprolactinaemia
    Anorexia nervosa
    Psychogenic amenorrhoea
    Exercise-induced amenorrhoea
    Fertile eunuch syndrome

Hypergonadotropic hypogonadism
Gonadal dysgenesis
    Turner syndrome
    Klinefelter syndrome
    XX and XY gonadal dysgenesis
Other forms of primary gonadal failure
Disorders of gonadal steroidogenesis = congenital adrenal hyperplasia (CAH)
    Lipoid CAH
    17α-Hydroxylase/17,20-lyase deficiency
    3β-Hydroxysteroid dehydrogenase deficiency
    20,22-Desmolase deficiency

---

30 Primary amenorrhoea

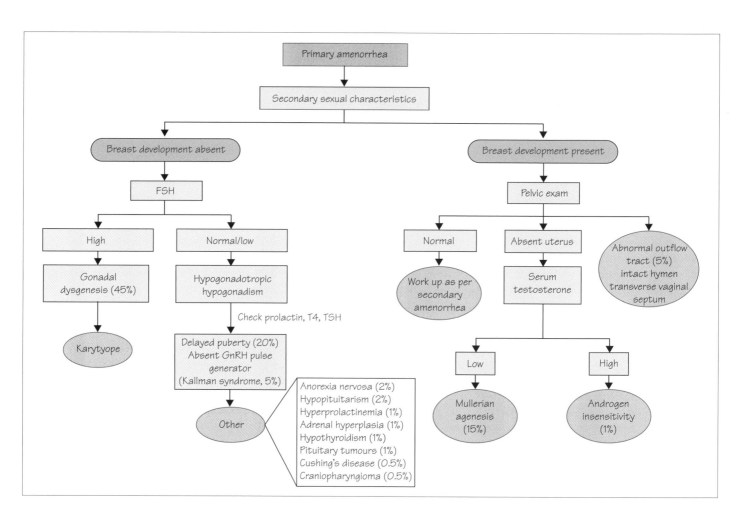

Overview

Primary amenorrhoea is defined as failure to menstruate by age 16 in patients with normal secondary sexual characteristics or the failure to menstruate by age 14 in patients with no signs of sexual maturation. **Secondary amenorrhoea** is defined as the absence of three menstrual cycles or the absence of menstrual bleeding for 6 months. The distinction between primary and secondary amenorrhoea has traditionally been emphasized because of the higher incidence of genetic and anatomic abnormalities among young women with primary amenorrhoea. It remains conceptually useful to make this distinction because of several unique disorders that are found only in patients with one or the other. Still, there is much more overlap in the origins and pathophysiology of the two entities than was originally appreciated. For example, Turner syndrome is a common genetic cause of primary amenorrhoea, yet some patients with Turner syndrome have sufficient ovarian reserve to undergo secondary sexual development and menarche before complete ovarian failure results in secondary amenorrhoea. Other young women with chronic anovulation due to functional disorders will be classified with primary amenorrhoea if the onset of the disorder occurs at puberty. In such cases, it may be more useful to assess the degree to which secondary sexual characteristics have developed in girls with absent menses. Failure of breast and pubic hair development is a sign of

delayed or absent puberty and represents a specific subset of reproductive abnormalities (Chapter 29).

As the table shows, causes of amenorrhoea are extensive and involve all levels of the hypothalamic–pituitary–gonadal–end-organ axis. To avoid confusion, amenorrhoea can be divided into two broad categories of abnormalities. The first and largest category is characterized by chronic anovulation. In these patients, a failure to generate cyclic ovarian oestrogen and progesterone leads to absent or highly irregular sloughing of an inappropriately stimulated endometrium (Chapters 11 and 15). Chronic anovulation results from four general pathophysiological mechanisms: (i) the hypothalamus fails to generate a cyclic gonadotropin-releasing hormone (GnRH) signal to the pituitary gland; (ii) the pituitary fails to respond to appropriate signals from the hypothalamus; (iii) the normal sex steroid feedback mechanisms fail to drive the midcycle luteinizing hormone (LH) surge; (iv) interference with gonadal steroid feedback by other endocrine systems. The second, much smaller, category includes end-organ abnormalities that interfere with the ability of these organs to respond to normal cyclic ovarian steroid production and produce visible endometrial bleeding.

Diagnosing the underlying cause of amenorrhoea involves sequential determination of the function of each of the potentially affected compartments (uterus and vagina, ovaries, pituitary and hypothalamus).

Treatment aims to correct the underlying dysfunction so that menses resume. If it is not possible to establish or restore menstruation, it is very important to assess the hormonal status of untreated or inadequately treated individuals. Chronically hypoestrogenic women are at increased risk for osteoporosis (Chapter 24) and women with chronic unopposed oestrogen stimulation of their endometrium are at risk for endometrial cancer (Chapter 42). Hormonal therapy to avoid these consequences must be considered in all amenorrhoeic women.

Aetiologies of primary amenorrhoea

These are best understood if categorized by: (i) the presence or absence of breast development; (ii) the presence or absence of the cervix and uterus; and (iii) circulating follicle-stimulating hormone (FSH) levels. The figure opposite presents an algorithm for evaluating the girl or woman with primary amenorrhoea. Unsurprisingly, abnormalities in each of the four compartments mentioned above can be associated with primary amenorrhoea.

In order of descending frequency, the most common causes of primary amenorrhoea are gonadal dysgenesis, physiological delay of puberty, Müllerian agenesis, transverse vaginal septum or imperforate hymen, Kallman syndrome, anorexia nervosa and hypopituitarism. Complete androgen insensitivity, while much rarer than Müllerian agenesis, must be considered in any young woman who has breasts but no uterus. All girls or women with primary amenorrhoea and an elevated FSH must have a karyotype performed to determine if a Y chromosome or even a piece of a Y chromosome is present. The presence of any Y chromosome genes and an intra-abdominal gonad, regardless of its phenotype, confers a risk for germ-cell tumour development. These gonads must be surgically removed, typically at the time of diagnosis.

Gonadal dysgenesis with a pure 45X karyotype can usually be diagnosed because of the other physical features of Turner syndrome (Chapters 27 and 29). Other abnormalities of the sex chromosomes can also cause amenorrhoea, including 45X/46XX, other mosaics, and 46XY with a missing SRY locus (Chapter 6). **Müllerian agenesis**, also known as the Mayer–Rokitansky–Kuster–Hauser syndrome, is characterized by a complete absence of the female internal genitalia, including the vagina, uterus and Fallopian tubes, in a chromosomally normal female. Its biological cause is unknown. **Transverse vaginal septa** are thought to result from failure of the vaginal plate to resorb at the site where the Müllerian ducts fuse with it to form the cervix (Chapter 27). **Kallman syndrome** is a developmental abnormality of the central nervous system (CNS) in which those neurosecretory cells destined to become the GnRH pulse generator fail to migrate from their origins in the olfactory placode to the median basal hypothalamus (Chapter 29). In addition to reproductive abnormalities, individuals with Kallman syndrome also cannot smell because of the absence of the olfactory neurons that develop from the same anlagen. **Anorexia nervosa** and the consequent hypothalamic suppression can cause delayed or absent puberty if the disorder begins in childhood, primary amenorrhoea if it begins during puberty, or secondary amenorrhoea if it begins later in adolescence. **Hypopituitarism** most commonly results from CNS tumours and can present as either absent or delayed puberty or amenorrhoea depending on timing of onset and the rate of tumour growth. **Complete androgen insensitivity (AI)**, previously called **testicular feminization**, is a rare X-linked disorder caused by mutations in the androgen receptor that make it unresponsive to androgen. Although they can make testosterone and other androgens, patients with complete AI cannot exhibit androgen activity at central or peripheral target tissues. Genitalia fail to masculinize during embryogenesis and androgens cannot exert negative feedback on FSH production by the pituitary gland. Individuals with complete AI are phenotypic girls and will develop breasts at puberty because the androgens secreted by their overstimulated testes can be converted peripherally to oestrogens. They do not have a uterus. Therefore, they will not menstruate and will present with primary amenorrhoea in the presence of adequate breast development.

Causes of amenorrhoea

Hypothalamic disturbances
Primary hypothalamic lesions
    Kallman syndrome
Secondary hypothalamic lesions
    CNS tumours
Abnormal CNS-hypothalamic interaction
    Anorexia nervosa
    Exercise-induced amenorrhoea

Primary pituitary disturbances
Sheehan syndrome (pituitary apoplexy)
Pituitary adenomas
Pituitary tumours
Empty sella syndrome

Secondary pituitary disturbances
Inappropriate gonadal steroid feedback
    Pregnancy
    Contraceptive steroids
    Constant oestrogen exposure
    Oestrogen excess
    Oestrogen-producing tumours
    Aromatase excess
    Oestrogen deficiency
    Gene mutations in oestrogen receptor
    Aromatase deficiency
    Androgen excess
    Androgen-producing tumours
    Functional excess (adrenal or ovarian)
Inappropriate feedback from other sources
    Polycystic ovary syndrome (PCOS)
    Cushing syndrome
    Hypo- and hyperthyroidism
    Lactation
    Hyperprolactinaemia
    Growth hormone excess
    Malnutrition

Gonadal abnormalities
Gonadal failure
    Gonadal dysgenesis
    Menopause
    Ovarian ablation or removal
Gene mutation in LH and FSH receptors

End-organ abnormalities
Uterus
    Müllerian agenesis
    Surgical removal of the uterus
    Endometrial ablation
    Asherman syndrome
Vagina
    Imperforate hymen
    Vaginal septum
Other
    Complete androgen insensitivity (testicular feminization)

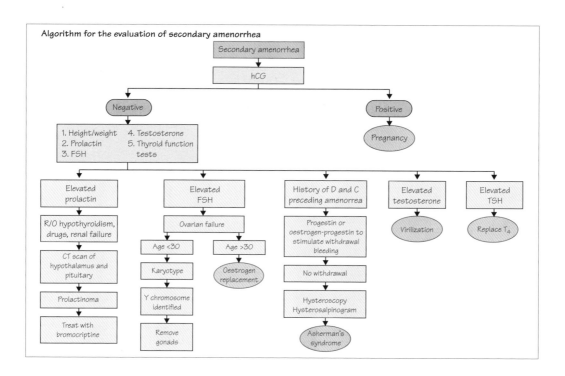

The aetiologies of primary and secondary amenorrhoea often overlap. Those more commonly associated with primary amenorrhoea are discussed in Chapter 30. Most secondary amenorrhoea results from anovulation. The most common reason is **pregnancy**; this aetiology should be evaluated before considering any other cause. An algorithm for evaluating secondary amenorrhoea is shown above.

Polycystic ovary syndrome (PCOS) is the most common cause of chronic anovulatory amenorrhoea. It is a disorder characterized by amenorrhoea or oligomenorrhoea, physical signs of hyperandrogenism (hirsutism, acne) and the presence of enlarged polycystic ovaries. PCOS pathophysiology can be linked to the combination of: (i) exaggerated pulsatile GnRH secretion, causing elevated circulating luteinizing hormone (LH) and an increased LH/FSH (follicle-stimulating hormone) ratio and (ii) defects in insulin signalling for glucose transport and lipolysis, causing insulin resistance.

The mechanism for the exaggerated GnRH pulse frequency and amplitude is unknown, but its appearance at puberty suggests an intrinsic, primary pathogenic defect. Pituitary gonadotrophs are exquisitely sensitive to the frequency and amplitude of GnRH pulses and the pattern present in PCOS patients causes a relative increase in the secretion of LH with respect to FSH. Ovarian theca cells respond to LH by increasing cholesterol conversion to androgens (Chapter 3). Conversion of these androgens to oestrogen in the ovary is reduced by a decrease in aromatase activity that accompanies the relative FSH deficiency. Hyperandrogenism, in turn, causes local follicular arrest and anovulation and systemic stimulation of sex steroid-responsive hair follicles, resulting in hirsutism and acne. The androgen-producing theca cells in the ovaries of PCOS patients become hyperplastic and are surrounded by an increased number of developmentally arrested primary and secondary follicles, which can be documented ultrasonographically as enlarged ovaries encircled by a 'string of pearls'.

Insulin abnormalities are as important in PCOS as those in the GnRH pulse generator. In fact, therapy with insulin sensitizers can correct both metabolic and hormonal alterations. In untreated patients, cellular defects in glucose transport result in transient hyperglycaemia and reactive hyperinsulinaemia. Insulin synergizes with LH to stimulate androgen production by theca cells and inhibits the hepatic production of sex hormone-binding globulin (SHBG), thereby increasing circulating free androgen. The cellular lipolytic defect in PCOS women results from a reduction in β-adrenoceptor density on adipocytes and causes increased fat storage and obesity. Obesity, present in over half of women with PCOS, amplifies the abnormalities of insulin resistance and hyperinsulinaemia.

The somatotropic (growth) axis has also been implicated in PCOS pathogenesis. Growth hormone (GH) and its peripheral mediators, insulin-like growth factors (IGFs), their binding proteins (IGFBPs) and their receptors enhance steroidogenesis by ovarian theca and granulosa cells. Non-obese PCOS patients have exaggerated GH pulse amplitudes, similar to their exaggerated GnRH pulses. In contrast, obese women with PCOS have hyperinsulinaemia but blunted GH secretion. Because insulin interacts with the IGF system at multiple levels and can bind to the IGF-1 receptor, hyperinsulinaemia mimics GH excess. In either case, there will be increased somatotropic activity and excessive androgen production in the ovary.

At least 50% of women with PCOS also show functional adrenal hyperandrogenism, making differentiation of PCOS from late-onset congenital adrenal hyperplasia (CAH) difficult. The exact nature of the adrenal dysfunction in PCOS is unclear, but evidence points to an increase in P450c17 activities in the zona reticularis of the adrenal cortex. LH, insulin and IGF-1 stimulate this same enzyme in the ovary to produce

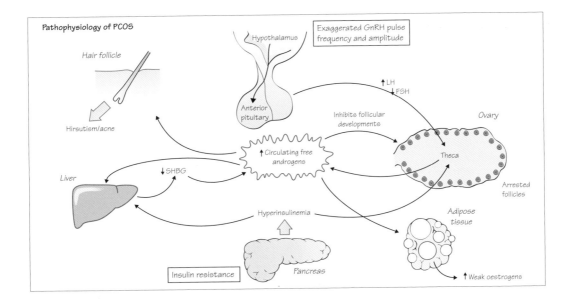

Pathophysiology of PCOS

androgens. PCOS patients with functional adrenal hyperandrogenism have exaggerated adrenal androgen production in response to adreno-corticotropic hormone (ACTH) stimulation. Excessive adrenal androgen production during adrenarche may trigger the onset of PCOS in these women by increasing serum androstenedione that is converted extra-gonadally to the weak oestrogen oestrone. Inappropriate oestrone production, in turn, may produce a premature and pathological trophic effect on the reproductive axis, causing PCOS at puberty.

Treatment of PCOS aims to reduce insulin resistance, to establish ovulation when fertility is desired, and to prevent prolonged unopposed oestrogen activity during anovulation and its associated risk for endometrial hyperplasia and cancer. Anti-androgens may be required to treat acne and hirsutism caused by hyperandrogenism.

All **functional hypothalamic disorders** are associated with decreased GnRH pulse frequency and amplitude. CNS input to the GnRH pulse generator can be disrupted by the psychogenic starvation of anorexia nervosa, by strenuous exercise and by stress. Infiltrative diseases of the hypothalamus like lymphoma and histiocytosis, while rare, can also disrupt GnRH secretion.

Amenorrhoea resulting from **excessive prolactin secretion** can arise from multiple abnormalities, including prolactin secreting micro- and macroadenomas, hypothyroidism and use of a wide variety of medications (Chapter 32).

Premature ovarian failure (POF), the cessation of menses before age 40 in the absence of genetic abnormalities, accounts for 10% of the cases of secondary amenorrhoea. Women with POF typically exhibit amenorrhoea, elevated gonadotropin levels and decreased circulating oestrogens. Many will have hot flashes. In most cases, the exact cause for ovarian failure will not be found. Some cases of POF are associated with autoimmune diseases such as Hashimoto thyroiditis, Addison's disease, hypoparathyroidism and myasthenia gravis, and may be part of a polyendocrine syndrome. Antibodies to gonadotropins and gonadotropin receptors have been found in some patients. Others lack antibodies, but carry genetic mutations in LH or FSH receptors. Occasionally, ovarian failure is temporary and pregnancies have followed an apparent cessation of ovarian function.

Intrauterine synechiae or adhesions occlude the uterine cavity in **Asherman syndrome**. Because the condition may develop after a postpartum curettage for heavy bleeding or infection, it is thought that these procedures can inappropriately remove deep endometrial layers and destroy the basal crypts and glands necessary for endometrial regeneration. The scarring associated with Asherman syndrome can totally obliterate the uterine cavity, although milder degrees of scarring can also cause amenorrhoea. Direct injury and local paracrine dysfunction may both be involved.

Hypothyroidism is associated with menstrual irregularities and amenorrhea. Thyroxine can increase oestrogen and progesterone secretion by cultured human granulosa cells and thyroid hormone deficiency may adversely alter ovarian steroidogenesis. Also, the increased hypothalamic secretion of thyrotropin-releasing factor (TRF) accompanying primary hypothyroidism will stimulate prolactin secretion. The resulting hyperprolactinaemia inhibits pulsatile GnRH secretion and causes menstrual irregularities (Chapter 32).

Congenital adrenal hyperplasia (CAH), Cushing syndrome and **obesity** all are associated with excess androgen production. Although adrenal androgens (DHEA and DHEA-S; Chapter 3) are relatively weak, their presence in pathological amounts can lead to significant androgenic effects. Most effects occur after conversion to more potent androgens and oestrogens in peripheral cells such as adipocytes. In women, the resultant non-cyclic, gonadotropin-independent sex steroid secretion interferes with normal cyclic secretion of FSH and LH by the pituitary and causes oligo- or anovulation.

In **empty sella syndrome**, the bony structure surrounding the pituitary gland is flattened and appears enlarged and empty. Some patients with an apparently empty sella will have headaches and no endocrine dysfunction. Others will have single or multiple endocrinopathies including gonadotropin deficiencies and hyperprolactinemia. The cause of empty sella syndrome is unknown.

The pituitary gland is particularly vulnerable to **hypotensive injury during pregnancy**. Pituitary infarction associated with postpartum haemorrhage and shock is called **Sheehan syndrome**. In Sheehan's original description, patients presented with panhypopituitarism. Such severe forms of Sheehan syndrome are rarely encountered in modern obstetric practice, but partial forms occasionally are. The severity of the injury determines the specific pituitary functions affected and loss occurs in a fairly predictable order. Most vulnerable is GH secretion. More severe cases will impair, in decreasing order of frequency, prolactin, TSH and ACTH secretion.

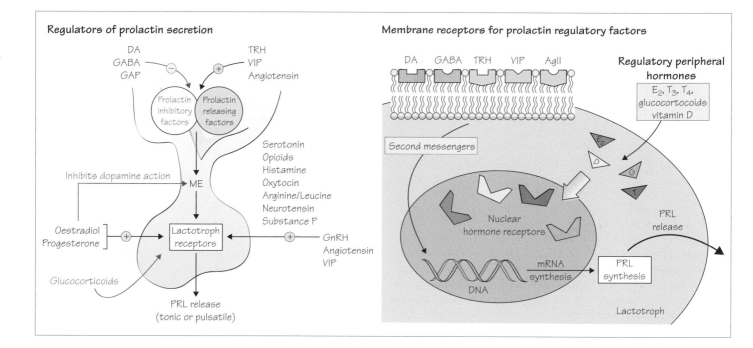

Regulators of prolactin secretion

DA
GABA
GAP

TRH
VIP
Angiotensin

Prolactin inhibitory factors

Prolactin releasing factors

Serotonin
Opioids
Histamine
Oxytocin
Arginine/Leucine
Neurotensin
Substance P

Inhibits dopamine action

ME

Oestradiol
Progesterone

Lactotroph receptors

GnRH
Angiotensin
VIP

Glucocorticoids

PRL release
(tonic or pulsatile)

Membrane receptors for prolactin regulatory factors

DA GABA TRH VIP AgII

Regulatory peripheral hormones

E_2, T_3, T_4, glucocortocoids vitamin D

Second messengers

Nuclear hormone receptors

DNA

mRNA synthesis

PRL synthesis

PRL release

Lactotroph

Hyperprolactinaemia is a common clinical problem. Cases resulting from inappropriate prolactin secretion by the pituitary gland are the third most frequently diagnosed cause of chronic anovulation and secondary amenorrhoea. There are many aetiologies for this condition; some result from serious underlying pathology and others from reversible functional disorders.

Control of prolactin secretion is dominated by tonic inhibition and there is no regulation by classic negative feedback from its target organs (Chapter 1). These characteristics are unique among pituitary hormones. The major inhibitor of prolactin secretion is dopamine and the two major stimuli are oestrogen and thyrotropin-releasing hormone (TRH). Numerous other neurohormonal regulators must be considered when elucidating the mechanisms by which hyperprolactinaemia develops.

Regulation of prolactin secretion

Embryonic differentiation of the lactotroph is under the control of the pituitary-specific transcriptional factor Pit-1. While Pit-1 regulates prolactin gene transcription by binding directly to the prolactin promoter, other regulators of prolactin gene expression use alternate pathways. Dopamine released into the pituitary portal system binds to a G_1 protein-coupled receptor and inhibits adenylate cyclase and phospholipase C. Acting as a neurohormone, rather than a neurotransmitter, dopamine reduces prolactin synthesis and prolactin release by the pituitary lactotrope. TRH acts through a second lactotroph cell membrane receptor to activate phospholipase C. In contrast to dopamine, TRH increases prolactin gene transcription and release of prolactin hormone from its storage granules. The effect of TRH is modulated by thyroid hormone such that decreases in T_3 and T_4 enhance prolactin release and increased concentrations of T_3 and T_4 decrease prolactin secretion. Oestradiol acts through a third mechanism, binding not to a membrane receptor but

to a nuclear receptor. The hormone receptor complex then interacts with oestrogen response elements upstream of the prolactin gene. Oestradiol also interferes with dopaminergic activation of its receptor and increases the concentration of TRH receptors on lactotrophs. Both actions potentiate the stimulatory effects of the sex steroid.

Like dopamine, γ-aminobutyric acid (GABA) and glucocorticoids inhibit prolactin secretion. The mechanism by which GABA acts as a prolactin inhibitory factor is unknown. Like oestrogen, glucocorticoids act through nuclear receptors to inhibit prolactin gene transcription. Vasoactive peptide (VIP), oxytocin, angiotensin II (AgII) and serotonin all increase prolactin secretion. VIP employs two mechanisms: it stimulates oxytocin release via the hypothalamus and it interferes with dopamine inhibition of adenylate cyclase. AgII acts on a specific membrane receptor on the lactotroph to provoke rapid release of presynthesized prolactin. It is a more potent secretagogue for prolactin than TRH. Serotonin released by the dorsal raphe nucleus also stimulates prolactin release but not its synthesis. Here, serotonin activity occurs independent of dopamine pathways.

In the physiological state, fine tuning of prolactin secretion is determined by the balance between the prolactin inhibitory factors (PIF) and the prolactin-releasing factors (PRF). Any disorder that alters the balanced secretion of these regulatory compounds will result in altered prolactin secretion. Regardless of its cause, hyperprolactinaemia can interfere with hypothalamic–pituitary function and result in hypogonadism with or without galactorrhoea. The fact that women with prolactin-induced amenorrhoea are hypo-oestrogenic but do not experience hot flashes suggests that one mechanism by which prolactin alters hypothalamic–pituitary function is via modulation of central neurotransmission. The hypothalamic dopaminergic and opioid systems that regulate gonadotropin-releasing hormone (GnRH) pulsatility are likely to be involved in this effect.

Physiological hyperprolactinaemia

Most physiological hyperprolactinaemia is transient and of no clinical consequence. High physiological concentrations of plasma prolactin occur at night and result from both an intrinsic circadian rhythm and sleep-entrained prolactin release. High protein meals at midday, but not in the morning, induce prolactin release through an unknown mechanism. Physical and emotional stress, including exercise, hypoglycaemia and anaesthesia are associated with elevations in prolactin secretion. Orgasm promotes prolactin secretion, but only in women. Pregnancy is associated with a marked elevation of prolactin secretion that persists into the immediate postpartum period (Chapter 23). Of all the physiological hyperprolactinaemic states, only lactation is associated with amenorrhoea.

Pharmacological hyperprolactinaemia

Medications that interfere with dopaminergic inhibition of the pituitary lactotroph can cause hyperprolactinaemia. Any drug that decreases the synthesis of dopamine, enhances its metabolism, increases its re-uptake or interferes with its binding to its receptor will reduce the action of dopamine. When the inhibitory activity of dopamine on the pituitary lactotroph is blocked, prolactin secretion increases. All of the medications listed in the table below can inhibit dopamine action and cause hyperprolactinaemia. Clinical manifestations of pharmacological hyperprolactinaemia include galactorrhoea and menstrual irregularities. Menstrual dysfunction may be severe enough to result in amenorrhoea.

Pathological hyperprolactinaemia

Lesions in the hypothalamus or in the pituitary gland may cause hyperprolactinaemia. Those in the hypothalamus typically do so by interfering with dopamine delivery to the pituitary gland. Tumours are the most frequent of the pituitary causes of hyperprolactinaemia; the prolactin-secreting adenoma is the most common of these. Prolactin-secreting adenomas (prolactinomas) are classified by size: microadenomas are less than 1 cm in size and macroadenomas are greater than 1 cm. These tumours can occur in both men and women, but are more common in women. In women they cause galactorrhoea, amenorrhoea, headache and visual field defects. In men they cause headache, visual field changes and impotence. They are often larger at diagnosis in men than in women because symptom onset is typically late in men.

Prolactinomas are usually benign. Pituitary adenomas that produce adrenocorticotropic hormone (Cushing disease) and growth hormone (acromegaly) may also cause hyperprolactinaemia.

Primary hypothyroidism can also cause hyperprolactinaemia. The decrease in circulating thyroid hormone that accompanies thyroid gland dysfunction diminishes negative feedback on the hypothalamus and pituitary gland. This results in an increase in TRH and TSH secretion. Excessive TRH can override the normal dopamine-dominated inhibition of prolactin secretion through direct, receptor-mediated effects on the pituitary lactotroph. A significant proportion of patients with chronic renal failure will have hyperprolactinaemia. While the aetiology of this effect remains incompletely described, patients with chronic renal failure appear to have circulating serum factors that interfere with dopaminergic inhibition of prolactin synthesis and secretion.

Treatment of hyperprolactinaemia is directed toward correction of the underlying cause. A notable exception to this rule involves the management of the prolactin-secreting pituitary adenoma. Resection of these tumours is associated with a high frequency of recurrence of the hyperprolactinaemia. Medical management is typically safer and more effective and involves use of oral dopamine agonists (e.g. bromocriptine). It is important to remember that men and women with hyperprolactinaemia are hypogonadal due to the associated abnormalities in the hypothalamic–pituitary–gonadal axis. This hypogonadal state places them at significant risk for osteoporosis (Chapter 24) and requires continuation of therapy for as long as the hyperprolactinaemia persists.

Galactorrhoea

Galactorrhoea describes the secretion of breast-milk in states unassociated with nursing. Galactorrhoea can result from hyperprolactinaemia or from excessive sensitivity of the breast to normal circulating levels of prolactin. If galactorrhoea is associated with amenorrhoea, then hyperprolactinaemia is likely the cause. If galactorrhoea occurs in the presence of normal ovulatory cycles, then excessive sensitivity of the breast to normal circulating amounts of prolactin is more likely. The three most common causes of hyperprolactinaemia resulting in galactorrhoea are (i) a pituitary adenoma, (ii) medications interfering with dopamine action and (iii) hypothyroidism. Galactorrhoea can be suppressed by the use of dopamine agonists.

Conditions associated with increased prolactin secretion

Physiological causes		Pharmacological causes		Pathological causes	
Sleep	Oestrogen therapy	CNS dopamine depleting agents		Hypothalamic lesions	Pituitary tumours
Feeding	Anaesthesia	Methyldopa		Craniopharyngioma	Cushing disease
Exercise	Dopamine receptor blockers	Monoamine oxidase inhibitors		Glioma	Acromegaly
Stress	Domperidone	Reserpine		Granulomas	Prolactinoma
Coitus	Haloperidol	Opiates		Histiocytosis	Non-secreting adenomas
Menstrual cycle	Metoclopramide	Stimulators of serotonergic system		Sarcoid	Neural reflexes
Pregnancy	Phenothiazine	Amphetamines		Tuberculosis	Chest wall injury
Postpartum	Pimozide	Hallucinogens		Pituitary stalk transection	Herpes zoster neuritis
Nursing	Sulpride	Histamine H$_2$ receptor antagonists		Head injury or postsurgical	Upper abdominal surgery
Fetal/neonatal		Cimetidine		Irradiation damage	Hypothyroidism
		Ranitidine		Pseudocyesis	Renal failure
		Nizatidine			Ectopic production
		Famotidine			Bronchogenic carcinoma
					Hypernephroma

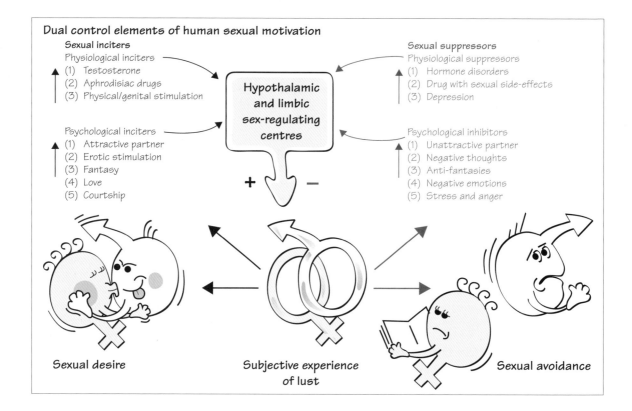

Prior to 1980, sexual dysfunction of any cause was lumped under the term 'impotence' for men and 'frigidity' for women. Since then, the classification of sexual disorders has evolved and is now based on the physiologically oriented, four-phase model of human sexuality (Chapter 16). This classification divides the sexual dysfunction syndromes into disorders of desire, disorders of excitement/arousal and disorders of orgasm. The fourth phase of the human sexual response, resolution, is rarely disturbed. Sexual desire disorders include hyper- and hypoactive sexual drive (libido) and sexual aversion. Excitement phase disorders include erectile dysfunction, dyspareunia and vaginismus. Orgasmic disorders include inhibited orgasm in women and premature ejaculation in men.

Sexual desire disorders

Normal sexual drive can be thought of as a balance between an 'erotic motor,' which incites a desire for sexual activity, and a 'sexual brake,' which keeps these urges in check. These excitatory and inhibitory signals appear to converge upon specific centres in the hypothalamus and limbic system to produce a continuum of sexual desire. It is probably only the polar ends of this continuum that are abnormal. There is no specific test for abnormal sexual desire. Instead, the diagnosis of a sexual desire disorder is based on the subjective reporting of abnormal libido that results in individual distress or interpersonal difficulty.

The two formally recognized sexual desire disorders are hypoactive sexual disorder (HSD) and sexual aversion disorder. HSD is defined as persistently or recurrently deficient (or absent) sexual fantasies or desire for sexual activity. Sexual aversion disorder is the persistent or recurrent extreme aversion to, and avoidance of, all (or almost all)

genital sexual contact with a sexual partner. Of patients seeking treatment for sexual desire disorders, 79% have HSD, 20% have sexual aversion disorder and 1% have hyperactive sexual desires. The causes of sexual desire disorders may be either organic or psychosocial. Organic causes include testosterone deficiency, chronic illness, certain centrally acting medications and underlying psychiatric disturbances. Psychogenic causes involve psychologically repressive stimuli such as anxiety, anger, perception of a partner as repulsive, or previous negative sexual experiences.

Treatment of the sexual desire disorders is directed first toward evaluation and correction of any underlying organic problem. Psychotherapy may be useful in the treatment of sexual desire disorders of non-organic aetiologies. Patients with long-standing sexual dysfunction of organic aetiology often develop concomitant psychosocial issues. Individual or group counselling may be extremely useful as adjunctive therapy in these patients.

Erectile dysfunction (impotence)

Erectile dysfunction (ED) is the recurrent inability of a man to get and keep an erection sufficient for intercourse. ED is mild if a man can usually get and keep an erection, moderate if he can only can get or keep an erection sometimes and complete if he never can. Risk factors for ED include aging, chronic illnesses, a variety of medications and cigarette smoking. It is a pervasive problem among older men; recent estimates report that 50% of 40–70-year-old men have some degree of ED. Even more are affected after the age of 70.

ED can occur because of vasculogenic, neurogenic, hormonal or psychogenic problems. Eighty per cent of the diagnosable conditions leading to ED are organic. They include, in decreasing order of frequency, atherosclerosis, diabetes, hypertension, medication side-effects, prostate surgery, hyper- and hypothyroidism, hyperprolactinaemia and hypogonadism. While depression is present in 60% of men with ED, it is often unclear whether this mood disorder is the cause or the result of long-standing ED.

Successful penile erection involves the activity of autonomic nerves upon the vascular smooth muscle of the penis. Relaxation of penile vascular smooth muscle allows blood to flow into the penis. Here it remains trapped and erection occurs (Chapter 14). Most of the organic causes of ED involve neuropathies of the autonomic nervous system, vascular compromise or, occasionally, testosterone deficiency. Psychogenic ED involves abnormal central inhibition of the erectile mechanism in the absence of demonstrable physical abnormality. Drugs that produce ED are myriad and typically affect the neural reflex pathways necessary for integrating the erection. Examples of medications associated with ED include antidepressants, antipsychotics, sedatives, antianxiety medications, antihypertensives and anticonvulsants. Alcohol and street drugs, including amphetamines, cocaine, marijuana, methadone and heroin, can also cause ED.

Until recently, treatment options for ED were limited to medication changes, implantable erection devices, intracavernosal injections of prostaglandins and psychotherapy. The discovery that the drug sildenafil can facilitate and maintain erections in impotent men has changed the treatment of ED dramatically. Sildenafil was originally tried as an antiangina medication and found to be ineffective. The study subjects were reluctant to turn in their leftover pills and soon the drug's unexpected side-effect was uncovered. Since then sildenafil, and related drugs, have been shown to be effective in the treatment of ED and have become widely available for this use. These medications work by inhibiting phosphodiesterase type V (PDE5), a cyclic guanosine monophosphate (cGMP)-metabolizing enzyme found predominantly in the penis. Nitric oxide (NO) activates guanylate cyclase in the penis, increasing cGMP, the major mediator of the vascular relaxation necessary for penile erection. The longer cGMP stays around, the longer the erection. Blockade of cGMP metabolism promotes and maintains NO pro-erectile activity. PDE5 inhibitors will not cause erections in the absence of sexual stimuli.

Premature ejaculation

This is a disorder characterized by ejaculation that occurs with minimal sexual stimulation after penetration and before the man wishes it. This must occur on multiple occasions over time to warrant diagnosis. When making the diagnosis, the man's age, the novelty of the sexual partner and circumstances and his frequency of sexual activity must be taken into account. Premature ejaculation is reported by 10–35% of men seeking help for sexual dysfunction. Unlike ED, which increases with age, premature ejaculation decreases with age.

The exact cause of premature ejaculation is unknown. The only demonstrable physiological correlate of premature ejaculation is that men reporting this disorder ejaculate at a lower level of sexual arousal than do control men.

Retrograde ejaculation

In men with retrograde ejaculation, semen travels backwards into the bladder rather than out of the penile shaft during ejaculation. The bladder neck does not close appropriately after emission and the cause is invariably organic. Neurological dysfunction is the most common mechanism underlying retrograde ejaculation. The three most common causes of such neurological dysfunction are: damage to penile innervation during prostate surgery, diabetic neuropathy and the use of anticholinergic medications. Retrograde ejaculation does not require intervention unless fertility is desired.

Dyspareunia

Patients with dyspareunia experience recurrent or persistent genital pain before, during (the most common) or after sexual intercourse. Of women seeking help with sexual problems 10–30% report dyspareunia, while only 1% of men report the problem. Because dyspareunia is reported so much more frequently in women than in men, much more is known about its aetiologies and interventional approaches in women.

Dyspareunia may reflect a physical or psychogenic problem. Details of whether the symptoms are lifelong or acquired, generalized or situational are helpful in identifying the potential aetiology. Organic causes of dyspareunia include the presence of hymeneal remnants, pelvic tumours, endometriosis, pelvic inflammatory disease, and vulvar vestibulitis. Hypo-oestrogenic states associated with menopause, the early postpartum period, use of very low dose oral contraceptives and prior treatment with chemotherapy may also cause dyspareunia. Psychosocial problems that result in dyspareunia may include poor self-esteem, poor body image, guilt and prior sexual abuse or trauma. Interpersonal factors between the couple, including anger, distrust and inadequate communication, may also be responsible.

Treatment of dyspareunia is directed toward evaluation and correction of any underlying organic problem. Psychotherapy may be useful in the treatment of dyspareunia of non-organic aetiology. It may also be useful as concomitant therapy for those with primary organic causes.

Vaginismus

Women with vaginismus experience recurrent involuntary spasms of the pelvic muscles of the outer third of the vaginal barrel, of such severity that intercourse is painful or impossible. Typically these occur in anticipation of intercourse or during penetration. In some women with severe vaginismus, spasms can also occur during a pelvic examination or tampon insertion.

Vaginismus occurs in 0.5–5% of women. There are significant intercultural differences. Lifelong vaginismus is a rare clinical entity in North America and most of Western Europe. It is relatively common in Ireland, Eastern Europe and Latin America. It is the most commonly reported cause of unconsummated marriages.

Like dyspareunia, vaginismus can have either an organic or psychosocial aetiology. The organic bases of the disorder are the same as those of dyspareunia. In fact, most experts believe that vaginismus begins as dyspareunia and escalates to vaginismus through a classical conditioning process. In this view, a woman first has pain on intercourse (unconditioned stimulus) and this leads to a natural self-protecting tightening of the vaginal muscles (conditioned response). Over time, stimuli associated with vaginal penetration can become conditioned stimuli and provoke the conditioned reflex muscle spasms. In severe cases, conditioned stimuli can even include thoughts of sexual intercourse.

Not all cases of vaginismus are classically conditioned from an organic cause. Many psychosocial contributors have been suggested, including guilt, religious constraints, responses to a partner's sexual dysfunction, prior sexual trauma, concerns about sexual orientation and fears of pregnancy, sexually transmitted diseases and trauma.

Like dyspareunia, treatment of vaginismus is directed toward evaluation and correction of any underlying organic problem, and psychotherapy.

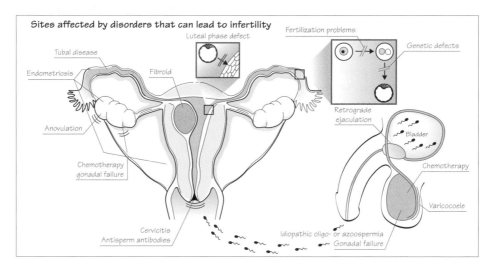

Infertility is defined as a diminished capacity to conceive and bear a child. It is not equivalent to sterility, the absolute and irreversible inability to conceive. Clinically, a couple is considered infertile if they are unable to conceive after 12 months of unprotected, frequent coitus.

Many factors contribute to infertility. Diseases that affect only females account for about one-half of infertile couples and diseases that only affect males about one-third. About 10% of couples will have disorders in both the male and the female partner. Some 10–15% of couples have no identifiable cause for their infertility or will become pregnant during the evaluation. Specific disorders causing infertility include those involving each of the major physiological events necessary to produce a pregnancy: (i) production of a healthy egg; (ii) production of healthy sperm; (iii) transportation of the sperm to the site of fertilization; (iv) transportation of the zygote to the uterus for implantation; (v) successful implantation in a receptive endometrium; (v) presence of other conditions, often immunological, that can interfere with one or more of the other events.

Oocyte abnormalities

The main cause of female infertility due to oocyte abnormalities is a failure to ovulate regularly or, in some cases, at all. Those disorders that result in oligo-ovulation or anovulation are also causes of amenorrhoea (see Chapters 30 and 31), and fall into three categories: hypothalamic dysfunction, pituitary disease and ovarian dysfunction.

Common hypothalamic causes of anovulation include abnormalities of weight and body composition, strenuous exercise, stress and travel. Pituitary or endocrine disorders associated with anovulation are hyperprolactinaemia and hypothyroidism. The two most common causes of ovarian dysfunction are polycystic ovary syndrome and premature ovarian failure. Oocyte abnormalities more complex than simple anovulation cause the decline in fertility that occurs as women enter their 40s.

Female anatomical abnormalities

Fallopian tubal disease is usually the result of inflammatory scarring of the Fallopian tubes. This may be caused by pelvic inflammatory disease, appendicitis with rupture, septic abortion, previous surgery and,

occasionally, previous use of an intrauterine device. The most common site of tubal blockage is the distal fimbriated end of the tube. These blockages are typically associated with additional pelvic adhesions and may affect up to 20% of the women in infertile couples. Purposeful, surgically induced blockage occurs with surgical sterilization; some women regret their contraceptive decision to have post-tubal ligation and present to the fertility specialist requesting reversal. **Endometriosis** is a common disorder, characterized by the presence of tissue resembling endometrium outside of its normal position lining the uterus. The glands and stroma of endometriosis are usually responsive to gonadal hormones and the biochemical changes the steroids induce in this ectopic endometrium mimic those seen in endometrium within the uterine cavity. Increased prostaglandin production by perimenstrual and menstrual endometriotic lesions is thought to promote the inflammation, fibrosis and adhesion formation characteristic of the disorder. Endometriosis lesions can be found almost anywhere in the pelvis but are most common on the peritoneal surfaces covering the pouch of Douglas, bladder, ovaries, Fallopian tubes, bowel and appendix. Women with endometriosis can present with pelvic pain, adnexal masses (endometriomas), infertility, or any combination of these.

Uterine **leiomyomas**, also known as fibroids or uterine myomas, are benign smooth muscle tumours of the uterus. They are the most common pelvic tumour in women, and may be located anywhere within the wall of the uterus or may hang from a stalk containing the blood supply to the tumour (pedunculated leiomyomas). Pedunculated leiomyomas may hang from the outside of the uterus or may project into the endometrial cavity. Those leiomyomas that distort the uterine cavity (submucosal in location) or physically obstruct Fallopian tubes are most closely associated with decreased fecundity.

Male factors

A **varicocele** is a dilatation of the pampiniform plexus of veins that drain the scrotum. Varicoceles appear to reduce semen quality in some men and their correction improves semen quality. The effect of correction on fertility is less clear. Varicoceles may adversely affect semen quality by exposing the testis to temperatures higher than those in non-affected men or by exposing the testis to abnormally high concentrations of gonadotoxic substances. Both effects appear to result from decreased venous efflux from the affected testis.

Blockage of the vas deferens or epididymis can result from congenital abnormalities [i.e. mutations in the cystic fibrosis transmembrane regulator gene (Chapter 26)], from infection-associated scarring, or from inadvertent surgical ligation at the time of inguinal surgery. Purposeful, surgically-induced blockage occurs with vasectomy; some vasectomized men regret their contraceptive decision and present to the fertility specialist requesting reversal.

Damage to the bladder neck or injury to the lumbar sympathetic nerves involved in the ejaculation reflex may cause retrograde ejaculation, as may neurological conditions such as multiple sclerosis if they inhibit normal innervation to the bladder neck. In this condition, sperm pass into the bladder upon ejaculation rather than exiting from the penile urethra. Therapy is unnecessary if fertility is not desired. If it is, medical therapies may augment bladder neck closure. If these fail, sperm may be harvested from alkalinized urine.

Men may also produce very few or no sperm because of inadequate hormonal stimulation of the testis or because of gonadal failure. Men with hypogonadotropic hypogonadism may have pituitary gland or hypothalamic defects (e.g. Kallman syndrome). They fail to secrete gonadotropins and so lack appropriate testicular function. These men are good candidates for treatment with exogenous gonadotropins. Most will respond and produce viable sperm. Men with gonadal failure [e.g. Klinefelter syndrome (47XXY)], have few therapeutic options. Some with oligospermia or azospermia will never discover the cause of their disorder.

Implantation abnormalities

Implantation abnormalities encompass a group of endometrial and embryonic defects that interfere with the complex communication occurring between these entities early in the post-conception period. Luteal phase deficiency (LPD) is the most discussed of the endometrial disorders that may directly impact implantation. LPD describes a group of endometrial maturation abnormalities that have been associated with subfertility and recurrent pregnancy loss. In LPD of ovarian aetiology, abnormal follicular development and ovulation lead to a relative deficiency in progesterone production. This delays or minimizes the effects of progesterone in converting the endometrium into a secretory organ receptive to implantation. Diagnostic tests for the condition are presently suboptimal.

Other factors

Many other factors can influence fecundity; a large proportion of these are immunological. Antisperm antibodies have been identified in some patients with infertility but have also been detected in fertile couples. Their aetiological role and treatment remain unclear. Inflammatory cells recruited into cervical mucus in response to cervical infections may affect sperm function, perhaps through release of cytokines. Some women develop antibodies against negatively charged phospholipids commonly encountered in cell membranes. These antiphospholipid antibodies can promote thromboses in small vessels leading to local ischaemia and infarction. Although antiphospholipid antibodies more typically result in recurrent early miscarriage, some women experience loss so early as not to know they are even pregnant. In these women, the antiphospholipid syndrome may initially manifest itself clinically as infertility.

Genetic abnormalities such as the androgen insensitivity (Chapter 26) and gonadal dysgenesis syndromes (Chapters 26 and 27) can also cause infertility. Gonadotoxin exposure, including exposure radiation and chemotherapeutic agents, can cause gonadal dysfunction and impaired fertility.

Evaluation and treatment of infertility

Evaluation initially involves assessment of the male partner with a semen analysis and documentation of ovulatory menstrual cycles and patent Fallopian tubes in the female partner. In some couples, additional testing will be indicated. This may include: anatomical assessment of the uterine cavity, evaluation of ovarian reserve by measuring serum FSH and oestradiol levels in the early follicular phase of the cycle, and, when indicated, a laparoscopy or hysteroscopy.

Once the evaluation is complete, treatment is directed by the findings. Anovulatory or oligo-ovulatory women are treated either by correction of any underlying problem such as hyperprolactinaemia or hypothyroidism or by induction of ovulation. Medications used for the induction of ovulation work by a variety of mechanisms. The most commonly used is clomiphene citrate, an oestrogen partial agonist/antagonist that acts at the level of the hypothalamus and pituitary gland to block oestrogenic negative feedback. This increases gonadotropin secretion. Aromatase inhibitors act to reduce circulating oestrogen levels, again blocking negative feedback centrally and promoting gonadotropin production and release. Both medications require a functioning hypothalamic–pituitary–ovarian axis. Patients who are not candidates for, or who fail the prior therapies can be treated with gonadotropin injections.

Reproductive tract surgery to remove endometriosis or a fibroid tumour may be recommended, although medical therapy for some of these problems is also available. In the past, tubal reconstructive surgery was a mainstay of infertility treatment; where readily available, assisted reproductive techniques like *in vitro* fertilization (IVF) have virtually eliminated the need for this approach.

Treatments for male factor infertility may first address the underlying aetiology directly. This may include medical or surgical therapies, such as correction of a varicocele or correction of blockage in the vas deferens. More commonly, assisted reproductive techniques are used to bypass sperm problems. Sperm can be washed, concentrated and placed directly into the intrauterine cavity using artificial insemination. The sperm source can be the woman's partner or a donor.

The widespread availability of the assisted reproductive technologies has revolutionized infertility treatment, making pregnancies possible under circumstances never before considered treatable. The most common treatment approach is IVF, in which multiple harvested oocytes are fertilized by spermatozoa in the laboratory. The resulting embryos are grown in the laboratory for 2–5 days, then a group of embryos are selected and transferred back into the cavity of the uterus. Standard IVF can be modified in a number of ways. Donor eggs or donor sperm can be used. In cases of severe male factor infertility, sperm can be injected directly into the oocyte cytoplasm to effect fertilization (intracytoplasmic sperm injection, ICSI). These sperm can be immotile. They can be retrieved directly from the vas deferens, epididymis, or even the testis in men with obstructive azospermia. Finally, recently developed technology allows genetic assessment of the embryos created through IVF. Using pre-implantation genetic diagnosis (PGD), a single blastomere is removed from a developing blastocyst. This blastomere can be screened for a variety of selected heritable single gene defects or for numerical chromosomal content. The results of screening can be used in selecting those embryos that will be transferred back to the uterus.

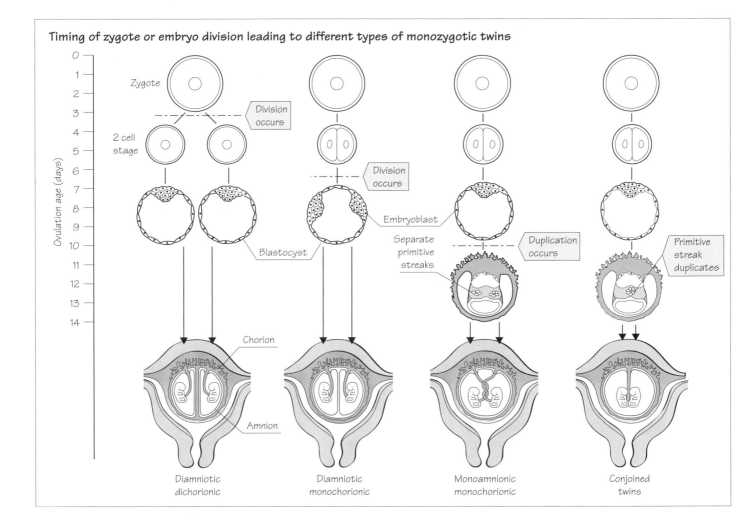

Timing of zygote or embryo division leading to different types of monozygotic twins

Overview

Twins may arise from one of two mechanisms, division of a single fertilized ovum into two embryos (**'identical' or monozygotic twins**) or fertilization of two separate ova (**'fraternal' or dizygotic twins**). Either or both processes may be involved in the generation of higher numbers of fetuses. Triplets could develop from one, two or three ova; quadruplets from one, two, three or four and so on. It is exceedingly rare for a zygote to divide more than once.

The two twinning processes have very distinct origins and implications for pregnancy outcome. While all multiple gestations carry a risk of preterm delivery from early labour, monozygotic twin pregnancies carry an additional risk of placental problems, chromosomal abnormalities and fetal malformations. These can dramatically influence pregnancy outcomes.

Biology of monozygotic twinning

It is not known exactly what causes an embryo to divide to produce monozygotic twins. However, it is clear that division of the fertilized ovum at specific early stages of development is responsible for the spectrum of clinical presentations with monozygotic twinning. These stages are depicted in the figure above. Basically, the earlier the fertilized ovum divides, the more separate the twins. Cleavage prior to development of an inner cell mass will result in two placentas, two sets of membranes and two fetuses, whereas division after the embryonic disk has formed results in conjoined twins.

The most common type of monozygotic twinning arises from division in days 3–8 after fertilization. This produces a pregnancy with two amniotic sacs and a single placenta (**diamniotic monochorionic twins**). The second most common type of monozygotic twinning results from a division of the embryo within the first 72 h after fertilization and produces a pregnancy with two amniotic sacs and two placentas (**diamniotic dichorionic twins**). Twins resulting from divisions later than day 8 after fertilization are rare. If the division occurs on or after the amnion forms on day 8 post-fertilization, both fetuses will be in the same amniotic sac (**monoamniotic monochorionic twins**). Siamese or **conjoined twins** are the rarest and arise from cleavage of the differentiating embryonic disk 13–16 days post-conception. Fraternal twins are always diamniotic dichorionic. Therefore, it is necessary to perform zygosity testing on twins with separate placentas who are suspected of being monozygous.

Aetiology of dizygotic twins

Most of the spontaneously conceived multifetal pregnancies are twin gestations. The incidence of conception of twins is at least twice the rate of liveborn twins. In many cases, one of a pair of diamniotic dichorionic twins just disappears. Less often, the whole pregnancy miscarries. The frequency of monozygotic twinning is about 1 set in every 250 births and is relatively fixed in most populations. In contrast to monozygotic twinning, the incidence of dizygotic twinning varies dramatically among different populations. Dizygotic twinning is highly influenced by race and heredity. Maternal age over 40, increasing parity and infertility treatment are positively linked to dizygotic twinning.

The racial differences in dizygotic twinning are quite marked. Twinning among Asians is least common, with a rate of only 1.3 dizygotic twin births per 1000 total births in Japan. White women in the USA and the UK have rates of about 8 dizygotic twin sets per 1000 births. Black women have the highest rates of all. They range from a rate of 11 per 1000 births in the USA to 49 per 1000 in some tribes in Nigeria, or 1 in every 20 births! The influence of heredity on dizygotic twinning is carried largely through maternal lineages, with about a 2% chance of delivering twins if the mother herself is a dizygotic twin. When the father of the baby is a dizygotic twin, the rate of twinning is only 0.8%.

In developed countries, most multifetal pregnancies result from infertility treatments. Ovulation induction, in vitro fertilization (IVF) and other assisted reproductive techniques dramatically increase the frequency not only of twinning, but also of conceiving higher order multiple gestations (triplets, quadruplets and more). The table below lists the most recent outcome data approximating the frequency of multifetal pregnancies in the United States, dependent on the means of conception. If one uses Hellin's theorem to calculate the expected frequency of twins in Nigeria, which has the highest spontaneous twinning rate in the world, one can see the impact of infertility treatment on the higher-order multiple gestations. Hellin's theorem states that if the frequency of twinning is n in a population, then the frequency of triplets is n^2, quadruplets n^3, and so on. Using $n = 0.05$ for the Nigerian tribes, one would only expect 0.25% triplet and 0.012% quadruplet gestations. Thus, infertility treatment can increase the risk of triplets 20-fold and quadruplets 80-fold over the world's most 'twinningest' people!

Although infertility treatment dramatically increases the frequency of non-identical multiples, the rate of monozygous twinning is also double that expected in these women. A disproportionate number of these monozygotic twins are also monochorionic. Transfer of day 5 blastocysts into the uterus during IVF is associated with a higher rate of monozygotic twins than transfer of day 3 zygotes. The stimuli for monozygotic twinning following ovulation induction alone have not been identified. Elevated gonadotropins promote recruitment of more than one ovarian follicle in a given cycle and represent the single most important risk factor for dizygotic conceptions. This is most evident during infertility treatments where the use of injected gonadotropins is associated with the development of multiple ovulatory follicles. The increased rates of spontaneous twinning seen with black race, advancing maternal age, parity and heredity are also related to elevations in endogenous gonadotropins, most notably in FSH.

Pregnancy risks with multiple gestations

The inherent risk in multiple gestations depends largely on whether single or multiple placentas are present and on whether there is a shared amniotic sac. All monochorionic twins have some degree of vascular connection within the placental bed. In about 15% of monochorionic twin pregnancies, these vascular connections permit the exchange of blood between the two fetuses. When this occurs, the haemodynamics of the two twins can become so deranged that one fetus will preferentially pump extra blood into the other (the so-called 'twin–twin transfusion syndrome'). The 'donor' twin becomes anaemic and produces an abnormally low amount of amniotic fluid, whereas the 'recipient' twin is volume overloaded and produces excessive amounts of amniotic fluid. Fetuses in multiple gestations also have an increased risk for abnormal insertion of the umbilical cord onto the placenta. The umbilical cord typically inserts into the middle of the placental disk and is completely surrounded by a protective layer of Warton's jelly. With multiple gestations, each fetus has an increased incidence of having a cord insert along the edge of the placenta (**velamentous insertion**). Cords with velamentous insertions are not completely surrounded by Warton's jelly and can be kinked or compressed more readily than more protected cords. Such compression can result in suboptimal fetal blood flow. The umbilical cords of monoamniotic twins invariably become entangled. This leads to fetal deaths in over half of the cases.

In addition to the problems that can arise from their placentas and membranes, monozygotic twins are also at increased risk of chromosomal abnormalities and congenital malformations. Because affected twin pairs are often discordant for the abnormality, it is presumed that whatever intrauterine events caused these embryos to divide can also randomly increase the risk for disordered embryonic development.

All multiple gestations are at risk for growth restriction of one or more of the fetuses. The risk increases as the number of fetuses increases. There are many possible causes for fetal growth restriction in multiple gestations. Suboptimal perfusion of the area of placental implantation of one or more fetus can cause fetal growth restriction. Velamentous umbilical cord insertions may also cause decreased fetal perfusion and growth restriction, as can donation of blood to a co-twin in the twin–twin transfusion syndrome.

All multiple gestations are at risk for preterm labour (Chapter 36.2). The risk increases in parallel with increasing numbers of fetuses. Uterine distension may explain the early onset of labour in pregnancies complicated by multiple gestations; however, other non-mechanical factors may also be involved.

Multifetal pregnancy rates using different infertility treatments (% of births)

Treatment	Twins	Triplets	Quadruplets +
None	1.2	0.015	0.00017
Aromatase inhibitors	3–4	<1	–
Clomiphene	8–10	<1	–
Gonadotropins	15	5	0.6
IVF	29	6	1

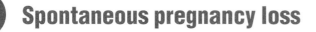

36 Spontaneous pregnancy loss

Miscarriage

A miscarriage is defined as a spontaneous pregnancy loss before 20 weeks of gestation, and the medical term is **spontaneous abortion**. Miscarriages occur in 15% of recognized pregnancies. The total number of human conceptions far exceeds the number of births. It is estimated that at least 60% of all human conceptions do not result in a viable pregnancy, with the majority of these being spontaneously lost before or shortly after an expected menses. These pregnancies can be documented by the appearance and disappearance of a pregnancy-specific hormone (hCG; Chapter 19) from the maternal bloodstream. It is clear that there is a sensitive and effective mechanism in the maternal system that can detect abnormal pregnancies and prevent survival of the overwhelming majority.

It is impossible to know the causes of those pregnancy losses that occur around the time of the expected menses, the so-called 'chemical pregnancies'. They probably result from a myriad of abnormalities and pregnancy loss represents the final common clinical outcome. Abnormalities may occur in the conceptus or in the microenvironment of the maternal reproductive tract at the time of conception. The latter may result from congenital or acquired anatomical defects in the uterus. They may also be caused by endocrine abnormalities that alter the maturation of the ova prior to ovulation, the development of the embryo during transit to the intrauterine cavity or the growth and maturation of the endometrium as it prepares for implantation.

It is known that the most frequent cause of overt miscarriage is a chromosomal abnormality in the conceptus. At least 60% of miscarriages have a gross chromosomal abnormality that can be detected in the expelled fetal material. The table below lists the frequency of specific chromosomal abnormalities in miscarried material. It is usually not possible to identify a specific aetiology for the remaining 40% of isolated spontaneous pregnancy losses, although some are the result of an underlying problem that can lead to recurrent pregnancy losses (see below).

Increasing maternal age is accompanied by an increase in the frequency of chromosomal abnormalities in embryos and fetuses and in the rate of spontaneous pregnancy loss. Age-related egg abnormalities are thought to account for the majority of this effect, consistent with the dramatic rise in spontaneous pregnancy loss that is seen among mothers who are 35 or older. This effect is not noted in association with paternal age until the father of the pregnancy has reached at least 55 or 60. Even then, the effect is more subtle. Interestingly, an increase in the frequency of certain psychiatric disorders among offspring is associated with paternal aging. Ovum deterioration is thought to explain most of the decline in fertility after the maternal age of 40.

Most spontaneous pregnancy losses are heralded by vaginal bleeding and a fall in maternal serum hCG during the first trimester of pregnancy. During the first 12 weeks of pregnancy, hCG normally rises with a doubling time of about 48–72 h. The hCG level will typically plateau or drop before tissue is passed in pregnancies with threatened miscarriages. Thus, it would appear that the common signalling mechanism for abnormal pregnancies may be a disruption in the expression of the hCG gene located on chromosome 19. How trisomies and other chromosomal aneuploidies produce this effect on the hCG gene is not known. Moreover, fetuses with trisomy 13, trisomy 18 and trisomy 21 (Down syndrome) can be carried to viability. It is equally puzzling how these three trisomies escape the hCG signalling surveillance. Trisomy 21 is actually associated with an increase in circulating hCG in the second trimester. This finding is used during the first trimester of pregnancy in serum screening regimens that determine Down syndrome risk.

Recurrent pregnancy loss

Because one in every six pregnancies will result in a miscarriage, it is not uncommon for a woman to experience one or more spontaneous losses during her pregnancy attempts. A woman who has had two consecutive spontaneous losses, but has never carried a pregnancy to full term, has a 35% chance of a loss in her next pregnancy. If a woman has successfully carried a pregnancy in the past, she will not reach a similar level of risk for spontaneous loss in a subsequent pregnancy until she has experienced three losses. For this reason, diagnostic work-up should be initiated in women with two losses if no successful pregnancies have occurred in the past. Clinicians may choose to wait until a third loss in patients who have had successful pregnancies. It is reasonable to consider initiating diagnostic testing at an earlier point in the clinical history among women with infertility or advanced maternal age.

Causes of recurrent pregnancy loss (recurrent miscarriage) include parental chromosome translocations; structural uterine abnormalities such as longitudinal septa and intrauterine adhesions; endocrine disorders, including luteal phase defects, polycystic ovary syndrome (PCOS), hyperprolactinaemia, thyroid dysfunction and poorly controlled diabetes mellitus; autoimmune conditions such as the antiphospholipid antibody syndrome and a variety of heritable thrombophilias. Couples experiencing recurrent pregnancy losses are appropriately anxious and should be evaluated for an underlying cause in the hope that a specific intervention may prevent future spontaneous pregnancy losses.

Preterm labour

Overview

Preterm labour is the onset of labour before 37 weeks of gestation. It is the final common pathway for a number of conditions that induce uterine contractions at a time when the uterus is normally quiescent.

Preterm labour complicates 7–10% of all pregnancies and is a very large contributor to perinatal morbidity and mortality. Although over half the cases of preterm labour occur without warning, some factors do carry an identifiable risk. These include multiple gestation, uterine anomalies, third trimester bleeding, intrauterine infection, excessive amniotic fluid volume, maternal smoking and a history of prior preterm delivery. There have been numerous unsuccessful attempts to use risk scoring, close clinical observation and home uterine contraction monitoring to predict women at high risk for preterm labour. Several biochemical markers suggest increased risk of preterm labour. These include increases in salivary oestriol, which reflects activation of the fetal hypothalamic–pituitary–adrenal axis and in cortisol-releasing hormone, which is synthesized by the placenta (Chapters 20 and 22). Fetal fibronectin is normally restricted to the fetal compartment but will appear in vaginal secretions of women who are at risk for preterm delivery. More importantly, the absence of fetal fibronectin in maternal vaginal secretions is highly predictive of women who will not experience preterm labour.

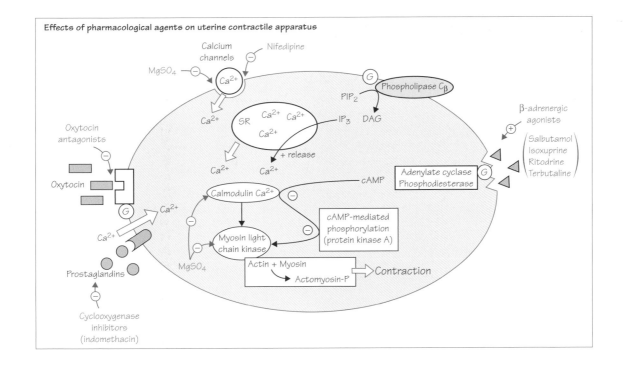

Effects of pharmacological agents on uterine contractile apparatus

Potential mechanisms for preterm labour

The normal mechanisms involved in labour (Chapter 22) predict the pathways for stimuli that start labour prematurely. For instance, intrauterine infection is associated with an elevation in the amniotic fluid levels of the cytokines interleukin-1β, interleukin-6 and tumour necrosis factor α (TNF-α). Products of the cyclo-oxygenase and prostaglandin pathways are also elevated in patients with intrauterine infections. Cytokines and prostaglandins act synergistically to stimulate the myometrium. Their premature elevation with intrauterine infection could activate the uterus prematurely. Recently, thrombin has been shown to be an extremely potent uterotonic agent. The increase in thrombin production that accompanies bleeding in pregnancy may cause preterm labour. Multiple gestations and excessive amniotic fluid excessively stretch the myometrial syncytium. While this may stimulate muscle activity, it is unclear how fibre stretching produces the regular, coordinated contractions of labour.

Pharmacological interventions

In some cases of preterm labour, contractions represent an attempt by the uterus to expel the fetus from a hostile intrauterine environment. This may be the goal when premature labour accompanies intrauterine infection. It is usually not prudent to intervene by attempting to stop labour in these clinical situations. When the cause of preterm labour does not independently place the fetus in danger, pharmacological attempts to stop the premature contractions may be used. Several agents, called **tocolytics**, are available to inhibit premature uterine contractions. Tocolytics work by interrupting one of four processes: (i) intracellular Ca^{2+} homeostasis; (ii) myosin phosphorylation; (iii) prostaglandin synthesis; or (iv) oxytocin binding to its receptors (see figure above). Calcium ions are required for normal myometrial contractions. Magnesium sulfate ($MgSO_4$) acts as a competitive antagonist for Ca^{2+} and is a commonly used tocolytic. High extracellular magnesium concentrations inhibit Ca^{2+} entry into myometrial cells via voltage-operated channels. In addition, intracellular magnesium competes with Ca^{2+} for binding sites on calmodulin. Decreased calcium/calmodulin

binding decreases the activity of myosin light chain kinase and muscle contraction. Nifedipine and nitrendipine are type II dipyridamole calcium channel blockers. They prevent Ca^{2+} influx through the cell membrane into the myometrial cells via the voltage-operated Ca^{2+} channels. β-Adrenergic agonists, such as ritodrine, salbutamol, isoxuprine and terbutaline, bind to $β_2$-adrenergic receptors on the myometrial cell membrane, activate G proteins and increase intracellular cAMP levels. An increase in cAMP levels activates protein kinase A. Activated protein kinase A inhibits myosin light chain phosphorylation. Prostaglandins E and $F_{2α}$ stimulate uterine contractions. The tocolytic indomethacin reduces prostaglandin production. It competitively inhibits cyclo-oxygenases that are necessary for conversion of arachidonic acid to prostaglandins. Oxytocin antagonists bind to the oxytocin receptor but do not activate it. Antagonist-binding blocks activation by the agonist oxytocin. Progesterone prophylaxis has been shown to reduce the rate of preterm birth among women with a history of spontaneous preterm delivery. The mechanism of action of the supplemental progesterone is not known.

Relative frequency of aberrations in chromosomally abnormal abortuses

Type	Incidence (%)
Trisomy	(52 total trisomy)
14	3.7
15	4.2
16	16.4
18	3.0
21	4.7
22	5.7
Other	14.3
45X	18
Triploid	17
Tetraploid	6
Unbalanced translocation	3
Other	4
Total	100

37 Pre-eclampsia

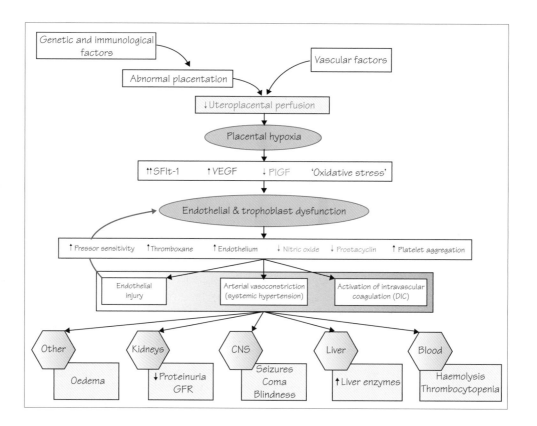

Clinical spectrum of pre-eclampsia

Pre-eclampsia is a unique disorder found only in human pregnancies. **Historically pre-eclampsia has been defined as the triad of hypertension, proteinuria and oedema** in a pregnant woman. **Eclampsia** is the occurrence of seizures that cannot be attributed to another cause in a patient with pre-eclampsia. Pre-eclampsia typically occurs in the third trimester of pregnancy, although some cases manifest earlier. Although many patients with pre-eclampsia demonstrate the classic triad above, it is now clear that the disorder is really a spectrum of clinical signs and symptoms that accompany microvascular changes in multiple organ systems. The disorder has so many presentations that it has been called the 'great imitator'. Central nervous system involvement can result in severe headaches, visual changes, seizures, stroke and blindness. Renal involvement is almost always present and can manifest as proteinuria, oliguria or renal failure. Oedema can accumulate in many sites, including the feet, hands, face and lungs. Haemoconcentration, thrombocytopenia and intravascular haemolysis are common signs of haematological involvement. Hepatic dysfunction often accompanies haematological changes and produces a group of clinical findings known as **HELLP syndrome** (**h**aemolysis, **e**levated **l**iver function tests, **l**ow **p**latelets). Patients with HELLP will often develop vague epigastric pain that may be mistaken for heartburn, gallbladder disease or the flu by an unsuspecting health care provider.

The overall incidence of pre-eclampsia in the obstetric population is 7–10%; the absolute number depends on the proportion of patients at increased risk. Risk factors for developing pre-eclampsia include the primigravid state (first pregnancy), multiple gestation, diabetes, pre-existing hypertension, a long interval between pregnancies, pre-eclampsia in a previous pregnancy, a family history of pre-eclampsia, hydatidiform mole, and inherited and acquired clotting disorders (e.g. protein S and protein C deficiencies and antiphospholipid antibodies). There is considerable overlap between the risk factors for pre-eclampsia and those for fetal growth restriction (FGR). Indeed, the presence of FGR may be the first sign of impending pre-eclampsia and women with pre-eclampsia are at risk for delivering a growth-restricted baby.

Left untreated, pre-eclampsia can be a highly morbid and even fatal disease. The ultimate treatment for the condition is delivery of the pregnancy. This is so effective a therapy that all deranged physiology will revert to normal after delivery provided that no permanent tissue damage has occurred. If the mother is medically supported through a timely delivery and postpartum recovery, her kidneys will begin to make urine again, blood will clot and seizures will stop. In spite of its potential for a 100% cure with proper diagnosis and treatment, pre-eclampsia remains one of the leading causes of maternal death in both developed and developing countries.

Potential mechanisms in pre-eclampsia pathogenesis

It is clear that the placental abnormalities are central to the pathogenesis of pre-eclampsia. Delivery cures pre-eclampsia and hydatidiform mole, a form of gestational trophoblast disease characterized by placental overgrowth but no fetal development (Chapter 44), predisposes to the disease. It was originally thought that the placenta secreted a toxin that that caused pre-eclampsia and the disorder was appropriately called **'toxaemia'**. While no unique toxins have been identified in the circulation of patients with pre-eclampsia, abnormal concentrations of specific metabolites are found in many of these patients. Circulating thromboxane, a vasoconstricting prostaglandin, is elevated while nitric oxide production is subnormal. Cytokines, placental fragments, free radicals and reactive oxygen species are also elevated in many of these patients. Most recently, a soluble form of a vascular endothelial growth factor (VEGF) receptor (sVEGFR-1 or sFlt-1) was shown to be markedly elevated in the serum of pregnant women weeks before the symptoms of pre-eclampsia become manifest.

Theories about the aetiology of pre-eclampsia abound, but no single mechanism has proven to be wholly responsible. It is likely that there are several initiators of the disease that ultimately converge in a final common pathway. Examination of the small blood vessels in the uteri of women with pre-eclampsia often reveals a failure of the invading trophoblast to appropriately remodel the spiral arteries (see figure below; cf. normal placentation, Chapter 18). There are several explanations for why the cytotrophoblast fails to properly invade these vessels. The necessary molecular conversion of the trophoblast from an epithelial cell type to an endothelial cell type may fail to occur. Cytotrophoblast differentiation into an invasive phenotype is accompanied by production of VEGF and a placental growth factor, PlGF. Placentas from pre-eclamptic pregnancies secrete increased amounts of sFlt-1, the soluble antagonist to VEGF. Excess sFlt-1 could inhibit or reduce the development of the invasive phenotype.

Pre-eclamptic women may suffer abnormal immune activation and this may inhibit trophoblast invasion of maternal blood vessels. This could explain why pre-eclampsia is most common when a woman is exposed to paternal antigens for the first time: a first pregnancy or, in a multigravid woman, the initial pregnancy with a new partner. Loss of immune tolerance over time would also explain why a long interval between pregnancies is a risk factor for developing pre-eclampsia. Abnormal activation of the immune system underlies other autoimmune diseases, such as systemic lupus erythematosus, that carry an increased risk for pre-eclampsia. The elevated serum cytokine levels detected in women with pre-eclampsia could also result from a primary immunological disorder.

Specific genetic abnormalities may be involved in the pathophysiology of pre-eclampsia. Women who carry a mutation in the complement receptor CR-1 have an increased risk for pre-eclampsia. Pre-existing insulin resistance confers an increased risk. The fact that a family history of pre-eclampsia increases a woman's risk for the disease indicates that there may be many more genetic predispositions to the disease.

A mismatch between fetal/placental demands and the maternal ability to meet them may cause pre-eclampsia and would explain risk factors such as multiple gestation, maternal vascular disease and hypercoagulable states. Proponents of this theory propose that the undernourished fetus sends signals to the mother to increase perfusion of the placenta. If the mother cannot compensate in response to the signal, the fetus sends more urgent signals. Pre-eclampsia results from the effects of excessive signals. As an example, hypoxia has been shown to increase the production of sFlt-1 by cytotrophoblast. Increased sFlt-1 may be part of the pathogenesis of pre-eclampsia.

While the initiating placental abnormality is unclear, the final common pathway for pre-eclampsia is known to be **endothelial dysfunction and injury**. The vascular endothelium normally functions to prevent microcoagulation and to modulate vascular tone. Vascular injury results in coagulation and alters the response of the underlying vascular smooth muscle to vasoactive substances. Often, substances that act as vasodilators on an intact endothelium will cause vasoconstriction of damaged endothelium. In pre-eclampsia, endothelial dysfunction can solely explain the basic triad: hypertension (vasospasm), oedema (capillary leak) and proteinuria (renal cell damage secondary to hypoperfusion). Experiments in animal models indicate that excess sFlt-1 can directly produce some of the organ dysfunction seen in pre-eclampsia. What remains inexplicable is why only a few, but not all, of the signs and symptoms of pre-eclampsia will appear in any given patient.

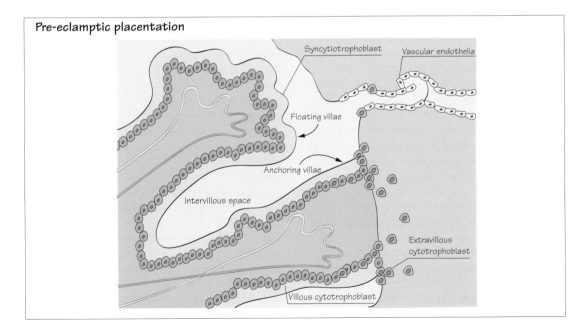

Pre-eclamptic placentation

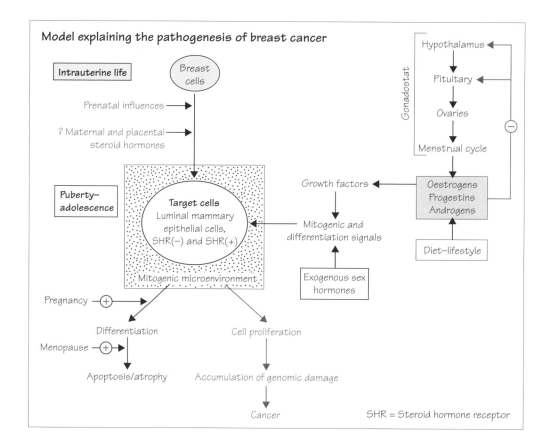

Model explaining the pathogenesis of breast cancer

Overview

Breast cancer is the most common malignancy in women. In addition to being predominantly a disease of women (99% of breast cancers occur in women), it is also a disease of aging. The lifetime risk of developing breast cancer is largely concentrated in the perimenopausal and post-menopausal years. The effect of aging on breast cancer risk is not widely known among the public; older women tend to underestimate their risk and many women under 50 years of age grossly overestimate their risk. Consequently, these two groups of women misjudge the benefits of breast cancer screening programmes.

Breast cancer may arise anywhere in the mammary gland. Tumours are typically classified by their cells of origin: lobular or ductal. Ductal carcinomas account for 85% of breast cancers and can be either non-invasive (intraductal) or infiltrating. Those ductal carcinomas that are histologically confined by the basement membrane of the duct are called intraductal carcinomas or ductal carcinoma *in situ* (DCIS). DCIS is considered a precursor lesion to invasive carcinoma. At least 33% of these lesions will progress to invasive cancer within 5 years.

Once the basement membrane of the duct is breached, an infiltrating carcinoma has developed. The most common type of invasive carcinoma is ductal carcinoma (no special type), accounting for 79% of invasive carcinomas. The next most common type is lobular carcinoma. These lesions arise from the terminal ductules of the alveoli and comprise approximately 10% of invasive breast cancers. Less common types of infiltrating carcinomas include medullary carcinomas, mucinous (colloid) carcinomas and Paget's disease. Paget's disease is a special subtype of infiltrating ductal carcinoma localized to a main lactiferous duct. In Paget's disease, eczematous changes develop in the nipple and areola overlying the affected duct. These skin changes are often the first sign of disease although the cancer may have been present for some time.

Breast cancer metastasizes first to the regional axillary lymph nodes. The most frequent distant metastatic sites are bone, liver, lung, pleura and brain. Patients with histologically negative axillary nodes have a much higher likelihood of survival than do patients with positive nodes. The ultimate prognosis for the disease depends on the size of the tumour, the number of involved lymph nodes and whether or not lymphovascular invasion (LVI) is present.

Treatment of invasive breast cancer is typically multimodal, but ultimately depends on the stage of the disease at the time of diagnosis. Surgical options include a modified radical mastectomy or lumpectomy with local irradiation. Ipsilateral axillary lymph node dissection is also typically performed. Women with positive lymph nodes will usually receive additional antineoplastic chemotherapy. Those with negative nodes will receive adjuvant chemotherapy if they have large primary tumours or LVI, because both confer a high risk of tumour recurrence. Tamoxifen is a medication with oestrogenic and antioestrogenic properties; it is the most widely used endocrine therapy for breast cancer. Before employing endocrine therapy, it is important to know the oestrogen and progesterone receptor status of the tumour because only receptor-positive tumours predictably respond to medications like tamoxifen.

Treatment of DCIS is controversial and includes mastectomy or wide local excision plus irradiation. Recurrence rates following excision plus radiation are approximately 10%; half of these are invasive.

Epidemiology of breast cancer

The epidemiology of breast cancer in women suggests that it is an endocrine disorder related to prolonged exposure to ovarian hormones. Ovarian hormones have been shown to increase the mitotic activity of mammary cells in culture. In addition to the factors listed in the table opposite, hormonal treatment in the form of postmenopausal hormone replacement therapy may contribute to a higher lifetime risk of breast cancer.

There are also large ethnic and geographical differences in the prevalence of breast cancer. Asian women born and raised in Asia have one-fifth the risk of developing breast cancer that American women have. The risk rises toward the American level if Asians live in the USA for two or more generations, suggesting an environmental or lifestyle influence on the disease. Even within a single large country, breast cancer incidence and mortality rates can vary by location. In more affluent areas, breast cancer rates are elevated. This may be related to delayed child-bearing among more affluent and better educated women. The association of alcohol intake with increased breast cancer risk suggests there is an environmental influence on its development.

Familial breast cancer

About 10% of breast cancer is familial. The clustering of breast cancers with ovarian cancers in many familial cases led to the discovery of two genes, *BRCA1* and *BRCA2*. Individuals with germ-line mutations in these genes are at high risk for the development of specific cancers. Current evidence indicates that 75% of inherited cases of breast cancer result from mutations involving *BRCA1* and *BRCA2*. Both *BRCA1* and *BRCA2* are tumour suppressor genes and both alleles must be abnormal before tumourigenesis will occur. The ethnic and geographic distributions of *BRCA1* and *BRCA2* are discussed in more detail in Chapter 41.

Molecular biology of sporadic (non-familial) breast cancer

Molecular studies have identified several genetic loci that are frequently abnormal in breast cancer specimens but not in normal breast tissues. The most commonly encountered abnormalities involve the oncogenes, *ERBB2* and c-*myc*, the tumour suppressor gene *TP53*, and telomerase. Both oncogenes are amplified or overexpressed in about 30% of breast cancers; telomerase activity is elevated in 80–90%. Breast tissue with *ERBB2* abnormalities appears to be resistant to the effects of the anti-oestrogen tamoxifen but more sensitive to standard chemotherapeutic agents. *TP53* abnormalities interfere with normal apoptosis, thereby making affected tumours more resistant to chemotherapy and radiation therapy.

Like most malignancies, breast cancer probably results from the effects of environmental triggers on genetically susceptible tissues. Genetic susceptibility may result from germ-line mutations like *BRCA1* and *BRCA2* or from abnormalities arising during intrauterine or pubertal differentiation. Environmental influences such as prolonged ovarian hormone exposure may increase mitogenesis in the breast, predisposing mammary ductal epithelium to further genomic damage and transformation from atypical benign cells to a malignancy. Other environmental influences such as pregnancy may enhance breast cell differentiation and reduce the risk of an abnormal response to normal growth factors.

Increasing odds: risk for women 20 years of age of developing breast cancer

By age of	Number diagnosed with cancer
25	1 in 19 608
30	1 in 2525
35	1 in 622
40	1 in 217
45	1 in 93
50	1 in 50
55	1 in 33
60	1 in 24
65	1 in 17
70	1 in 14
75	1 in 11
80	1 in 10
85	1 in 9
Lifetime	1 in 8

Determinants of breast cancer risk

Factor	Relative risk
Family history of breast cancer	
First-degree relative	1.8
Premenopausal first-degree relative	3.0
Postmenopausal first-degree relative	1.5
Premenopausal first-degree relative (bilateral breast cancer)	9.0
Postmenopausal first-degree relative (bilateral breast cancer)	4.0–5.4
Menstrual history	
Menarche before age 12	1.7–3.4
Menarche after age 17	0.3
Menopause before age 45	0.5–0.7
Menopause from age 45 to 54	1.0
Menopause after age 55	1.5
Menopause after age 55 with more than 40 menstrual years	2.5–5.0
Oophorectomy before age 35	0.4
Anovulatory menstrual cycles	2.0–4.0
Pregnancy history	
Term pregnancy before age 20	0.4
First-term pregnancy at age 20–34	1.0
First-term pregnancy after age 35	1.5–4.0
Nulliparous patient	1.3–4.0
Histological risk factors	
Atypical ductal hyperplasia	1.3–4.5
Atypical lobular hyperplasia	4.0
Lobular carcinoma *in situ*	5.4–12.0
Other	
Affluent vs. poor	2.0
Jewish vs. non-Jewish	2.0
Western hemisphere	1.5
Cold climate	1.5
Obesity + hypertension + diabetes	3.0
Moderate alcohol intake	1.3

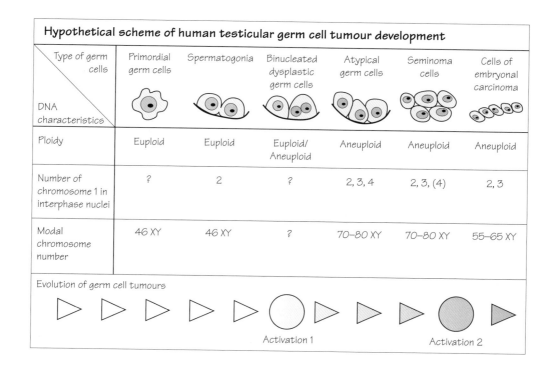

Hypothetical scheme of human testicular germ cell tumour development

Type of germ cells / DNA characteristics	Primordial germ cells	Spermatogonia	Binucleated dysplastic germ cells	Atypical germ cells	Seminoma cells	Cells of embryonal carcinoma
Ploidy	Euploid	Euploid	Euploid/ Aneuploid	Aneuploid	Aneuploid	Aneuploid
Number of chromosome 1 in interphase nuclei	?	2	?	2, 3, 4	2, 3, (4)	2, 3
Modal chromosome number	46 XY	46 XY	?	70–80 XY	70–80 XY	55–65 XY

Evolution of germ cell tumours

Activation 1   Activation 2

Overview

Testicular cancer is the most common malignancy in men in the 20–40-year age group. The germ-cell tumours (GCTs) are the most prevalent type of testicular cancer. Their incidence has risen over the past two decades, as has the most prevalent risk factor for GCT, an undescended testis (cryptorchidism). This suggests that the number of men afflicted with testicular cancer will continue to rise for the foreseeable future.

Unlike ovarian tumours, which are most likely to arise from the epithelium covering the gland, 90% of primary testicular tumours arise from intratubular germ cells. Histologically, there are six distinct types of GCT. Five of these occur in young men and one is seen exclusively in older men. The five subtypes seen in young men include **seminoma**, **choriocarcinoma**, **endodermal sinus tumour** (yolk sac carcinoma), **embryonal carcinoma** and **teratomas**, both benign and malignant. **Spermatocytic seminomas** are typically seen in men over 50 and are quite rare. The germ cells of origin in GCT affecting young and old men are distinct and appear to be at different stages of maturation. The associated tumours therefore have very different neoplastic behaviours.

All GCTs of young men arise from spermatogonial cells. The five tumours that develop from this single precursor cell type are quite heterogeneous and several exhibit embryonal-like differentiation. Prognosis and treatment depends upon whether GCTs are pure seminomas (SGCTs) or mixed cell tumours (non-seminomas, NSGCTs). Seminomas have a homogeneous germ-cell morphology. Non-seminomas have features of embryonal cells and can mimic the histogenesis of the very early embryo. Embryonal carcinoma is the most primitive, or pluripotent of the NSGCTs. It can progress along extraembryonic lines as choriocarcinoma or yolk sac carcinoma, or along embryonic lines as a teratoma. Individual tumours can contain a mixture of any of the histological subtypes.

About 80% of GCTs secrete tumour markers that can be detected in the serum. Tumours with yolk sac components typically secrete alphafetoprotein (AFP), an embryonic protein normally produced by the yolk sac during development. Other NSGCTs can also secrete AFP but seminomas do not. Human chorionic gonadotropin (hCG) is typically secreted by choriocarcinomas; however, small amounts of hCG production have been found in SGCTs as well as NSGCTs. The distribution of these two markers by specific cell types suggests the associated tumours arise from precursors at different levels of differentiation. AFP is a very primitive marker of embryonal differentiation whereas hCG represents trophoblastic differentiation. A third marker, placental-like alkaline phosphatase (PLAP), is found in carcinoma *in situ* (CIS) and about 50% of seminomas. Clinical paradigms using serum levels of AFP and hCG have been developed to assist in the diagnosis and staging of GCT.

Most GCTs are diagnosed at an early tumour stage when the tumour is confined to the testis. Serum screening, physical exam and testicular ultrasounds are useful in identifying early tumours in patients at high risk for GCT, such as formerly cryptorchid men and intersex individuals who keep their gonads. Men who present with solid testicular masses are usually treated by radical orchidectomy (removal of the testis). When GCT metastasizes, it typically spreads unilaterally to the para-aortic nodes. Distant metastases are generally found only in tumours with trophoblastic components.

Like gestational trophoblast disease in women (Chapter 44), GCT has a very high cure rate. Virtually all patients with early stage disease can expect to be cured. Initial treatment of stage I disease involves removal of the affected testes, followed by either abdominopelvic lymph node dissection, a short course of adjuvant chemotherapy or close surveillance. Even metastatic disease responds to chemotherapy with cure rates in excess of 90%.

Leydig cell tumours are a very rare form of testicular cancer (1–3%) and are associated with isosexual precocious puberty (Chapter 28).

Gonadal stromal tumours (sex cord-stromal tumours) include both Sertoli–Leydig cell and granulosa-theca cell tumours. They are extraordinarily rare in boys and men and are associated with phenotypic feminization.

Epidemiology of GCT

The single largest risk factor for GCT is cryptorchidism (Chapter 26). It is estimated that 2–3% of cryptorchid men will develop GCT, a relative risk 5–10 times that of the general population. GCT disproportionately affects white men of European descent and is uncommon in African and Asian men, independent of where they presently reside. Familial cases are also common. Pedigree analyses suggest that a single dominant gene with low penetrance is involved in these cases.

The strong developmental association of cryptorchidism with hormonal abnormalities suggests that fetal or neonatal endocrine imbalances may be involved in the initiation of GCT. The higher incidence of testicular cancer, cryptorchidism and hypospadias seen among the sons of women who were treated with the synthetic oestrogen diethylstilbestrol (DES) may provide mechanistic insights. Overexposure to oestrogens during fetal development may provide 'activation 1' leading to CIS formation with its aneuploidy and p12 abnormalities (see below). Increased levels of maternal oestrogen can suppress the fetal pituitary production of follicle-stimulating hormone (FSH) through negative feedback. Less FSH leads to reduced Sertoli cell multiplication and lower levels of Müllerian-inhibiting substance (MIS). Increased oestrogens may also impair Leydig cell function, thus decreasing local androgen production and testicular descent. MIS has been implicated as necessary for both normal descent of the testes and normal differentiation of fetal gonocytes into type A spermatogonia. Over the past 20 years, maternal oestrogen ingestion in the form of phyto-oestrogens (soya) and chemical pollutants with oestrogenic activity has increased, as has the incidence of both cryptorchidism and GCT.

Exposure of the cryptorchid testes to high temperatures may also play a role in the development of GCT, as the maturation of gonocytes to type A spermatogonia is significantly inhibited in abdominal testes. Still, maldescended testes that have been restored to the scrotum in infancy or childhood still retain an increased lifetime risk of GCT, as does the contralateral testis in cases of unilateral cryptorchidism. Heat exposure cannot be solely responsible.

Molecular biology of GCT

Because all GCTs have a sex chromosome constitution of XY, all tumours must originate in germ cells prior to the first meiotic division. These tumours are often aneuploid. Most common is a near triploid autosome content. Almost all GCTs exhibit multiple copies of chromosome 12p, either as one or more copies of i(12p) or as tandemly duplicated segments of 12p on marker chromosomes. These findings have led to the following model of tumourigenesis in GCT.

The precursor cell for GCT is the pachytene spermatocyte. These are the final premeiotic spermatogonial cells and therefore contain a 4C DNA content (Chapters 5 and 9). The homologous autosomes within these cells are paired as bivalents and the sex chromosomes are aligned. These chromosomes will cross-over and segregate as they progress to metaphase 1. The process of crossing-over requires activation of specific genes to repair the resulting open chromosomal ends. If the repair mechanisms fail, the affected spermatocyte degenerates. A meiosis stage cell with a defective repair mechanism is rescued from death only by the

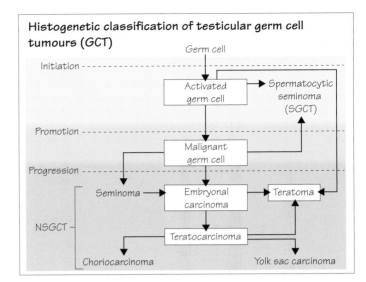

Histogenetic classification of testicular germ cell tumours (GCT)

initiation of a new programme for mitotic division. Such a proliferation is neoplastic. In the spermatocyte, the aberrant chromatid exchange event that initiates the new cell cycle must involve a locus on p12, given that it is almost uniformly abnormal in GCT. Aberrations in the p12 gene product appear to rescue the cell from death. Initiation of another round of DNA replication in the improperly repaired cell will lead to a tetraploid cell with an i(p12) or amplified p12. Because the initial repair defect remains, the cell is genetically unstable and more susceptible to additional chromosomal changes, such as non-disjunction, mutation and microdeletion.

It is not clear whether all GCTs derive from a single cell that has undergone malignant transformation (clonal expansion) or whether tumourigenesis can be multifocal. An alternative, but related, theory for GCT development hypothesizes that a subset of gonocytes undergo 'activation 1', during which they become bi- or multinucleated spermatogonia. Nuclear fusion occurs in some of these abnormal spermatogonia and they become tetraploid cells. These aneuploid cells then receive a 'second hit' or 'activation 2'. As a result, they lose specific genes or chromosomes that are important for tumour suppression. The clonality or multifocality of a given tumour might then depend on the nature of specific activating factors.

Regardless of how these cells undergo malignant transformation, it is clear that tumourigenesis can occur in infancy or even prenatally, perhaps as early as during testicular differentiation. Testicular CIS has been found in both fetal and neonatal testes. It is a polyploid non-invasive precursor to GCT that shares its aneuploidy and 12p amplifications. As the peak incidence of frankly invasive carcinoma occurs 2–3 decades after precursor lesions, GCT appears to have a very long latency, which supports the second hit or activation theory for the development of GCT. Early hormonal imbalances, particularly androgen exposure at puberty, may also play a role in the development of GCT, perhaps through the 'activation 2' step.

In contrast to GCT in young men, the spermatocytic seminomas seen in older men are more indolent and slow growing. Spermatocytic seminomas appear to arise from mature spermatogonia and not spermatogonial stem cells, which may explain their less aggressive behaviour. The molecular basis for such different biological behaviours may rely on imprinting (discussed further in Chapter 44).

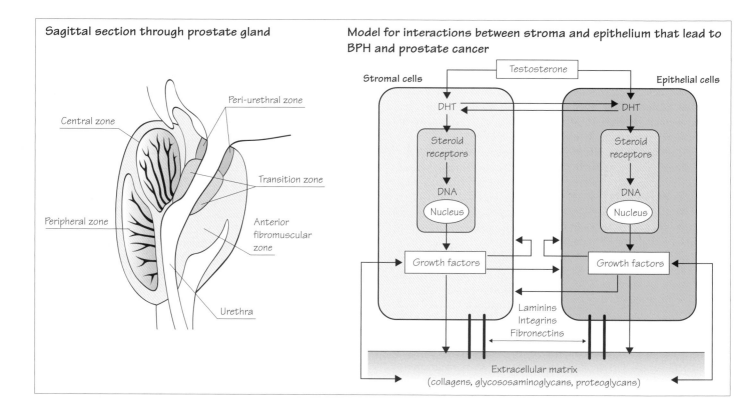

Sagittal section through prostate gland

Model for interactions between stroma and epithelium that lead to BPH and prostate cancer

Benign prostatic hypertrophy

Overview

The prostate is the organ of the body most frequently afflicted by disease in males over 50 years of age. The single most common pathological process is benign prostatic hypertrophy (BPH). At least 70% of 70-year-old men develop BPH; 40% suffer from some symptom of bladder outflow obstruction.

Epidemiology and symptoms

Age is a risk factor for BPH. Data suggesting that black race puts men at increased risk appear to be poorly controlled for socioeconomic status and access to health care.

BPH will cause urethral obstruction severe enough to warrant medical intervention in about 30% of elderly men. Interestingly, the overall size of the prostate does not correlate with either the presence or the severity of outflow obstruction. The fibromuscular hypertrophy that occurs with BPH can partially denervate prostatic and surrounding tissues, leading to urethral irritation and producing frequency and urgency of micturition, urge incontinence and nocturia.

BPH is characterized by a gradual increase in both the glandular and fibromuscular tissue in the peri-urethral and transition zones of the prostate that surround the urethra at its origin from the bladder and midsegment, respectively. Nodular hyperplasia is the characteristic microscopic change of BPH. It involves cellular hyperplasia plus associated changes in the architecture of the ducts and acini. Nodular hyperplasia of the peri-urethral zone consists of a mixture of glandular and fibromuscular elements, often with fibromuscular proliferation to the exclusion of the epithelium. Nodular hyperplasia in the transition zone is characterized by large amounts of glandular tissue that arise through budding and branching of pre-existing ducts. This latter type of hyperplastic proliferation is a highly unusual finding in adult human tissues, whether normal or diseased. It is felt that this anomalous development results from a reversion of the tissue to more embryonic behaviours.

Pathogenesis

The transition and central zones of the adult prostate gland appear to be of Wolffian duct derivation while the peripheral zone arises from the urogenital sinus (Chapter 7). These distinct embryological origins may explain why **BPH occurs within the transition and central zones** while prostatic adenocarcinoma originates within the peripheral zone.

The prostate glandular tissue is unique among the internal genitalia in that it requires dihydrotestosterone (DHT) for normal embryological development and for maintenance. Testosterone acts as a prohormone. It is converted locally to the more potent androgen DHT by 5α-reductase. DHT potency rests on the higher affinity of the prostatic nuclear androgen receptor for DHT than for testosterone.

Differentiation and growth of the prostatic epithelium is dependent on androgen-sensitive factors produced in the underlying stroma (embryological mesenchyme). Candidate growth factors increase mitosis in prostatic epithelial cells *in vitro* and include: epidermal growth factor (EGF), insulin-like growth factors (IGFs) and basic fibroblast growth factor (bFGF). Expression of bFGF is increased in BPH.

The development of BPH requires a normally functioning testis and the presence of functional 5α-reductase. Individuals lacking 5α-reductase have a vestigial prostate and never develop BPH or prostate cancer. Men with BPH have increased 5α-reductase activity and possibly an increase in prostate androgen receptors, making the 'ageing' prostate more susceptible to androgen stimulation. There may be a protective role for oestrogens in BPH. Oestradiol production slowly increases in older men when their testes become less responsive to luteinizing hormone (LH) so that more LH is required to maintain androgen production. High LH levels disproportionately stimulate oestrogen production. Elevated circulating oestrogens increase hepatic sex hormone-binding globulin (SHBG) synthesis and elevations in SHBG reduce the concentration of free testosterone in the circulation. This decreases the amount of testosterone available to be converted to DHT in the prostatic stroma.

Treatment of BPH

Treatment of BPH traditionally has been surgical resection via transurethral prostatectomy (TURP), the second most common operation performed in men over the age of 65 years. Medical treatment has focused on shrinkage of the prostate using 5α-reductase inhibitors and on symptomatic treatment of obstructive symptoms with α-adrenergic agents. The latter are effective because of the large proportion of smooth muscle containing adrenergic receptors in BPH.

Prostate cancer

Overview

Prostate cancer (PCa) is the most common non-cutaneous malignancy in the United States and Europe. It will certainly grow in frequency as the population ages. Autopsy series have consistently found incidental PCa in 15–45% of older men.

Epidemiology

Risk factors for PCa include age, race, positive family history, dietary fat intake, circulating hormone levels and possibly vasectomy. African-American men who consume a high fat diet are at the highest risk for Pca. Asian men residing in the Far East and subsisting on a low fat diet carry the lowest risk. Changes in geography or eating habits profoundly modify these background racial differences. Plasma androgen concentrations at the high end of normal increase PCa risk, as do SHBG or oestrogen concentrations at the lower end of the normal range. Obstruction of the vas deferens by vasectomy causes death of the seminiferous epithelium and Sertoli cells, leading to Leydig cell hyperplasia and increased local testosterone concentrations in the testicular veins.

As with most malignancies, PCa probably occurs as a result of environmental promoters in genetically susceptible tissues. For PCa, age and family history are predisposing factors and androgen is the promoter. Because the incidence of microscopic PCa appears independent of race and of geography despite markedly different incidence rates of clinically apparent disease, race may influence the progression of latent tumours to clinically evident tumours. Modest differences in androgen production among African-American, Asian and white men have been reported. These exposures over a lifetime may explain the influence of race on PCa.

The hereditary form is distinguished from the more common form by an earlier age of onset. Hereditary Pca is rare, although a positive family history confers significant risk for a given individual in that family.

Pathogenesis

Adenocarcinoma of the glandular epithelium of the peripheral zone of the prostate gland is the most common form of PCa. It results from androgen activity on a tissue that has acquired oncogenic potential. **Prostatic intraepithelial neoplasia (PIN)** is the earliest sign of an evolving neoplastic process. It is characterized by proliferation and anaplasia of the cells lining the ducts and glandular acini of the **peripheral zone** and disruption of the architecture of the basal epithelial cell layers.

Like most malignancies, the prognosis in PCa is determined by the stage and grade of the tumour at detection. Patients with disease localized to the prostate have an 80% survival rate at 5 years. The presence of distant metastases at diagnosis significantly lowers 5-year survival. PCa spreads locally to the hypogastric and presacral chains of lymph nodes and haematogenously to bone.

The interaction between prostatic stroma and epithelium appears to play an important role in the development of PCa. Different stromal growth factors are over-expressed in PCa when compared to BPH. Specifically, the stroma of PCa contains more IGF, EGF and TGF-β, while that in BPH contains more bFGF. DHT and testosterone both stimulate production of EGF and TGF-β by the prostate gland. The androgen dependence of these growth factors probably also accounts for much of the hormonal dependence of the normal prostate gland.

Mutations in the *ERBB2* oncogene cause increased EGF receptor (EGFR) activity in PCa. Similar *ERBB2* mutations are found in breast cancers. In both diseases, the EGFR shifts from its normal position in the basal epithelial layer to the luminal epithelium as the disease progresses from hyperplasia to intraepithelial neoplasia to frank cancer. Hereditary PCa is associated with mutations in the *BRCA1* or *BRCA2* tumour suppressor genes. Similar gene mutations are also associated with breast and ovarian cancers.

Loss of heterogeneity (LOH) studies have identified several chromosomal loci as potential sites for abnormal tumour suppressor activity in PCa. For instance, in PCa that metastasizes after therapy, there is a gain in genetic material at the site of the androgen receptor gene on the long arm of the X chromosome. The gene for the androgen receptor (AR) becomes amplified after androgen withdrawal treatment, an adaptation by the tumour that aids its survival under androgen-deficient conditions. This discovery sheds light on the molecular basis for the development of drug resistance by some cancer cells.

Prostate-specific antigen (PSA) is a protease secreted by the prostatic epithelium. Small amounts leak across the prostatic acini and into the plasma. PSA determinations have been used as a screening tool for PCa in asymptomatic men although the cost effectiveness of this approach remains unclear.

Treatment

Treatment of locally contained PCa utilizes surgery or irradiation. Irradiation combined with androgen ablation is reserved for widespread disease. Androgen withdrawal may be accomplished by orchidectomy, by treatment with a luteinizing hormone-releasing hormone (LHRH) agonist such as goserelin or leuprolide, or by treatment with an antiandrogen. Chemotherapy is not effective in treating Pca.

Ovarian neoplasms

Overview

The overwhelming majority of ovarian masses are benign and the life-time risk of developing ovarian cancer is about 2%. Age is the most important factor in determining risk of malignancy. Adnexal masses are common during the reproductive years. During this stage of life, such masses are usually caused by functional ovarian cysts, benign neoplasms of the ovary or by postinfectious changes in the Fallopian tubes. In girls under 20 and in women over 50, about 10% of all palpable ovarian masses are malignant. Between 85 and 90% of ovarian cancer occurs in postmenopausal women.

Benign neoplasms of the ovary

Benign and malignant neoplasms can develop from any cell type found in the ovary. Simple cysts can be functional and form at the site of ovulation or during the development of the corpus luteum. These are very common and distinguishable from true neoplasms by their transitory nature. They typically disappear within 6 weeks of discovery. Complex or solid masses and those that are persistent are more likely to be truly neoplastic and require histological diagnosis. Most benign neoplasms of the ovary are not premalignant lesions and will not progress to invasive cancer. Thus, careful screening and removal of benign and borderline tumours of the ovary during the last 20 years has not reduced the incidence of ovarian cancer.

Ovarian cancers

While over 90% of testicular malignancies are germ-cell tumours, 65–70% of ovarian malignancies are epithelial cell cancers. Germ-cell tumours of the testis have good early detection and high cure rates (Chapter 39). Ovarian epithelial cell cancers are usually detected after widespread intraperitoneal dissemination. At this point, cure is almost impossible

There are five distinct histological types of epithelial ovarian tumours: serous, mucinous, endometrioid, clear cell and Brenner. Of the five, serous neoplasms account for almost half of all tumours. Mucinous tumours comprise about 25%, endometrioid tumours about 5%, clear cell cancers under 5%, and Brenner cell tumours 2–3% of the total. The remainder of ovarian cancers are too poorly differentiated at diagnosis to be classified.

Epithelial ovarian cancer typically spreads both locally and by intraperitoneal dissemination. Contiguous spread is to the Fallopian tube and uterus. Dissemination occurs to the contralateral ovary and peritoneum. Implants of epithelial ovarian cancer may be found on the cul-de-sac, bowel, mesentery, omentum and diaphragm. Malignant ascites forms when diaphragmatic metastases block the lymphatic drainage of the peritoneal cavity. Patients with these cancers may not develop symptoms until the tumour mass compresses other intraperitoneal organs or the associated ascites causes abdominal bloating, dyspepsia or urinary frequency. This relative lack of early symptoms leads to late diagnosis and poor prognosis. Treatment for epithelial ovarian cancer involves cytoreductive surgery and aggressive chemotherapy, and only 15% of patients with advanced disease will survive. These tumours often develop resistance to chemotherapy. When disease is confined to the ovary, survival dramatically improves to 50–90%. Unfortunately, ovarian epithelial tumours are seldom diagnosed at this early stage.

About 15% of all epithelial ovarian cancers have histological and biological behaviours that are neither clearly benign nor frankly malignant. While these 'borderline' tumours have a 95% 10-year survival rate, they can recur as many as 20 years after excision. Late recurrences are often identical to the primary tumour, but malignant transformation to high-grade epithelial ovarian cancer is also seen, so it is unclear whether some borderline ovarian cancers are precursors to frankly malignant tumours.

Familial ovarian cancer

A variety of syndromes have been have been associated with increased risk for the development of cancers. Three include a predisposition to ovarian cancer: familial ovarian cancer syndrome, hereditary breast/ovarian cancer syndrome and Lynch cancer family syndrome II (hereditary non-polyposis colorectal cancer syndrome, HNPCC). These syndromes account for less than 10% of ovarian cancer diagnoses. Virtually all the hereditary breast/ovarian cancers and site-specific ovarian cancer syndromes are caused by mutations in the tumour suppressor genes *BRCA1* or *BRCA2*. Individuals with *BRCA1* mutations have a 20-fold increase in their risk for developing both breast and ovarian cancers, and those with *BRCA2* mutations a 5–10-fold increase in their risk for developing ovarian cancer. The estimated frequency of *BRCA1* mutations in the general population is 1/800, but is greater than 1/100 among Ashkenazi Jewish women. *BRCA2* mutations have a very similar carrier frequency among the Ashkenazi and a frequency of 1/250 among Icelanders.

HNPCC is caused by mutations in any one of three genes important in DNA mismatch repair. The most common extracolonic malignancy in women with HNPCC is endometrial cancer, followed by ovarian cancer.

Epidemiology of epithelial ovarian cancer

Family history is the most important risk factor, followed by age. The mean age of disease onset is 59 years. Other risk factors are early menarche, regular periods, short menstrual cycle length, low parity and a history of infertility. High parity and use of oral contraceptives reduce the risk of ovarian cancer. Both also decrease the number of lifetime ovulation events. These epidemiological data suggest that the number of ovulations over a lifetime is significant in the pathogenesis of the disease.

As with other prevalent epithelial cancers, environmental factors influence the development of ovarian cancers, with the highest rates being found in highly industrialized countries. Japan is the single notable exception, with rates of malignant neoplasms of the ovary that are among the lowest in the world. However, the rates in Japanese immigrants in the USA approach those of Caucasian natives within 2–3 generations, suggesting that carcinogens in the immediate environment are responsible. Chemical carcinogens from the outside world can reach the pelvic peritoneum of women through the vagina and upper reproductive tract. In fact, investigators have shown that more women with ovarian cancer use talc as a dusting powder on their perineum or sanitary napkins than matched controls. The association between talc and ovarian cancer is also biologically plausible. Talc is chemically related to asbestos and ovarian cancer is similar to the mesotheliomas that can develop after pulmonary exposure to asbestos.

Molecular biology of non-familial epithelial ovarian cancer

The typical advanced stage of epithelial ovarian cancers at clinical presentation, combined with the lack of identifiable precursor lesions for the more common serous and mucinous adenocarcinomas, make biological study of their development difficult. Some investigators believe that epithelial ovarian cancers arise in small inclusion cysts that develop when surface epithelial cells become entrapped in the physical defects left in the ovarian surface after ovulation. Others believe that the ovarian epithelium is a coelomic mesothelium that is more prone to metaplasia than other epithelia. Both theories are consistent with the epidemiological data, suggesting that events that disrupt the integrity of the ovarian capsule predispose to tumourigenesis.

As with other malignancies, ovarian cancer probably develops after multiple genetic 'hits' cause a cell to display invasive, neoplastic behaviour. One 'hit' typically involves activation of an oncogene and the second 'hit' involves the loss of one or more genes with tumour suppressor activity. Recurrent disruption and repair of the ovarian capsular epithelium and environmental insults that disrupt the coelomic mesothelium could lead to increased risk of activation of proto-oncogenes. *BRCA1* and *BRCA2* are tumour suppressor genes and inheritance of one abnormal allele makes 'second hits' a high statistical probability.

Several oncogenes have been identified with high frequency in non-familial cases of epithelial ovarian cancer. These include *ERBB2*, whose cellular homologue is the epithelial growth factor (EGF) receptor gene, and c-*fms* whose cellular homologue is the macrophage colony-stimulating factor (M-CSF) receptor gene. The most commonly found tumour suppressor abnormalities involve p53, the product of a tumour suppressing cell checkpoint gene located on chromosome 17p. Mutations in p53 occur in 50% of ovarian cancers, and allelic losses on chromosome 17p are found in up to 75%. Point mutations and loss of *PT53* are not found in benign or borderline ovarian tumours consistent with their lack of precursor status. Mucinous cancers of the ovary frequently show point mutations of the K-*ras* oncogene.

Endometrioid and clear cell cancers of the ovary, while rare, may be the exception to the rule that epithelial ovarian cancers do not have well-defined premalignant lesions. Both cancer types have been found nested within areas of endometriosis on the ovary. Furthermore, identical loss of heterozygosity (LOH) events have been detected in the cancer itself and in adjacent, non-transformed endometrial tissue. There is about a 1% risk of malignant transformation of ovarian endometriosis.

Other ovarian malignancies

Only 10% of ovarian cancers are germ-cell tumours (GCTs). These occur largely in girls and young women. Like GCTs in men, GCTs in women arise from immature germ cells and include five distinct histological types: **dysgerminomas**, **choriocarcinomas**, **endodermal sinus tumours** (yolk sac carcinomas), **embryonal carcinomas** and **teratomas**. The dysgerminoma is the female equivalent of the seminoma. GCTs of the testes are typically detected early in their development; GCTs of the ovary are not. For this reason, far less is known about GCT tumourigenesis in the female compared to the male (Chapter 39).

Benign ovarian teratomas are also known as **dermoids**. They represent a unique subclass of the female germ-cell tumours because they arise from more mature germ cells than the other GCTs. On gross examination, dermoids may contain hair, bone, cartilage and large amounts of greasy fluid that rapidly becomes sebaceous at room temperature. On histological examination, the tumours contain disarrayed clusters of many of the cell types normally seen in fetuses. Like other GCTs, the molecular event(s) that lead to activation of the germ cells in dermoids can occur *in utero* and benign ovarian teratomas have been detected in the fetus and newborn. These tumours display abnormalities in imprinting and are discussed in more detail in Chapter 44.

Stromal cell tumours are the rarest ovarian malignancies, accounting for 5% of the total. They may contain granulosa, theca, Leydig or Sertoli cells, and usually make large amounts of steroid hormones: granulosa or theca cell tumours make oestrogens and Leydig or Sertoli cell tumours make androgens. The occurrence of stromal cell tumours is not age dependent. Those secreting androgens can cause virilization while those secreting oestrogens can cause endometrial hyperplasia and irregular vaginal bleeding.

Histogenetic classification of ovarian neoplasms

Neoplasms derived from coelomic epithelium
Serous tumour
Mucinous tumour
Endometrioid tumour
Mesonephroid (clear cell) tumour
Brenner tumour
Carcinosarcoma and mixed mesodermal tumour

Neoplasms derived from germ cells
Teratoma
    Mature teratoma
        Solid adult teratoma
        Dermoid cyst
        Struma ovarii
        Malignant neoplasms secondarily arising from mature cystic teratoma
    Immature teratoma (partially differentiated teratoma)
Dysgerminoma
Embryonal carcinoma
Endodermal sinus tumour
Choriocarcinoma
Gonadoblastoma

Neoplasms derived from specialized gonadal stroma
Granulosa–theca cell tumours
    Granulosa tumour
    Thecoma
Sertoli–Leydig tumours
    Arrhenoblastoma
    Sertoli tumour
Gynandroblastoma
Lipid cell tumours

Neoplasms derived from non-specific mesenchyme
Fibroma, haemangioma, leiomyoma, lipoma
Lymphoma
Sarcoma

Neoplasms metastatic to the ovary
Gastrointestinal tract (Krukenberg)
Breast
Endometrium
Lymphoma

Endometrial cancer

Overview

Carcinoma of the uterine endometrium is the most common pelvic malignancy in women. The USA and Canada have the highest incidence rates in the world, whereas developing countries and Japan have incidence rates 4–5 times lower. Epidemiological data indicate that there are two forms of endometrial cancer. One is directly related to oestrogen exposure and is most common in the USA. The other is unrelated to oestrogen and occurs throughout the world. Oestrogen-related type I tumours occur among younger perimenopausal women and carry a good prognosis. In fact, type I lesions are potentially preventable through recognition of patient risk, diagnosis of the precursor lesion (atypical endometrial hyperplasia) and proper treatment. Non-oestrogen-related type II tumours occur in older postmenopausal women without a history of oestrogen exposure and have a poorer prognosis. The molecular genetic alterations present in type I and type II endometrial carcinomas are distinct and may help to explain their clinical characteristics.

Cells of the Müllerian tract can differentiate into a wide range of tissue types. This is demonstrated by the variety of histological subtypes seen among the endometrial cancers. The vast majority are endometrioid adenocarcinomas. Prognosis for patients with endometrioid adenocarcinoma is determined largely by its degree of differentiation or histological grade (well, moderately or poorly differentiated). In fact, histological grade is a prognostic factor independent of stage at diagnosis. Less common histological subtypes include mucinous adenocarcinoma, serous adenocarcinoma, clear cell adenocarcinoma, squamous cell carcinoma and a variety of rare mixed and undifferentiated tumours. For all subtypes other than endometrioid adenocarcinoma, prognosis depends more on histological subtype than on histological grade.

Endometrioid adenocarcinoma first invades the stroma of the underlying uterine tissue by destroying the glandular basement membrane. It then invades the myometrium and cervix. Endometrioid adenocarcinoma typically spreads via the pelvic and periaortic lymphatic channels rather than haematogenously. Vascular invasion is usually seen only with high-grade, non-oestrogen-dependent lesions.

Treatment of endometrial cancer usually involves surgical removal of the uterus, Fallopian tubes and ovaries. Patients with deep myometrial invasion or disease outside of the uterus may be treated postoperatively with radiation, chemotherapy or progestin-based hormonal therapies. Pretreatment analysis of endometrioid adenocarcinoma specimens for oestrogen and progesterone receptor status may help to direct postsurgical therapy. There is a good correlation between tumour differentiation and receptor content. Well-differentiated tumours usually have greater numbers of oestrogen and progesterone receptors. Because receptor content predicts response to progestin therapy, patients with well-differentiated tumours may be good candidates for progestin therapy.

The survival rate for endometrial cancer is relatively good. Overall, survival approaches 70% at both 5 and 10 years. Patients with stage I disease, in which the tumour has not invaded through more than half the myometrial thickness, have a 5-year survival rate of over 90%. Because of its high prevalence, endometrial cancer can be considered a neoplasia of high morbidity and relatively low mortality in developed countries.

Epidemiology of endometrial cancer

Endometrial cancer is largely a disease of the postmenopausal woman. About 80% of cases diagnosed are in women aged 50–75 years of age, with peak incidence in those aged 55–70. A woman entering menopause has double the chance of developing endometrial cancer compared with her chance for developing carcinoma of the cervix or the ovary. The incidence of endometrial cancer varies dramatically from country to country (see table below). This geographical pattern follows that of breast and ovarian cancer, with the highest rates in industrialized countries. It is exactly the opposite of patterns observed for cervical cancer.

An association between oestrogen exposure and endometrial cancer has been apparent for over 50 years. Many of the risk factors listed in the table on the next page are thought to increase the risk because of their close association with high oestrogen levels, typically unopposed by progesterone. The single most important and best-defined risk factor for adenocarcinoma of the uterus is obesity. Adipose tissue has active aromatase enzymes. Adrenal androgens are rapidly converted to oestrogens within the adipose tissue of obese individuals. These newly synthesized oestrogens also have excellent bioavailability because the metabolic changes associated with obesity inhibit the production of sex hormone-binding globulins by the liver. Obese individuals may have dramatic elevations in their circulating bioavailable oestrogens and this exposure can cause hyperplastic growth of the endometrium (see below).

Close links exist between the risk of endometrial cancer, a high fat diet and gross national product, which suggests that level of industrial development may affect incidence of endometrial carcinoma by influencing food consumption. A high fat diet is also associated with obesity and type II diabetes mellitus. Amount and type of dietary fat influences oestrogen metabolism. For example, diets rich in beef or in fats increase oestrogen reabsorption from the bowel.

White women are three times more likely to be diagnosed with endometrial cancer than black women. Again, this is exactly the opposite of what is seen for cervical cancer.

Steroid hormones and endometrial cancer

As noted above, the epidemiological data on endometrial cancer reveal a striking association between oestrogen exposure and cancer development. Interestingly, a direct causal link can only be inferred at this time. The basis for considering oestrogen as an aetiological factor comes from three sources: (i) the biological activity of oestrogen and progesterone on the endometrium; (ii) animal and human data on the effects of diethylstilbestrol (DES) on carcinogenesis; and (iii) the association of endometrial cancer with endometrial hyperplasia in conjunction with the association of hyperplasia with prolonged and unopposed oestrogen exposure.

The strongest attestation to the high sensitivity of the endometrium to ovarian steroid hormones is the dramatic changes that occur in this tissue during each menstrual cycle (Chapters 11 and 15). In a normally cycling woman, the endometrium changes its morphology on a day-to-day basis. In the follicular phase of the cycle, oestrogens stimulate proliferation of the epithelium covering the endometrial glands and of the underlying stroma. Oestrogen induces production of its own receptor and of the progesterone receptor during this time. Progesterone secreted after ovulation promptly arrests the proliferative activity in the glands and converts the epithelium to a secretory state. The stroma responds to progesterone with angiogenesis and functional maturation. If pregnancy should occur, these changes will prepare the endometrium for implantation. It is believed that the potent mitogenic effect of oestrogen on the epithelium of the endometrial glands accelerates the spontaneous mutation rate of predisposing oncogenes and/or tumour suppressor genes. This leads to neoplastic transformation.

Animal and human data gathered after developmental exposure to DES add biological evidence for the carcinogenic potential of oestrogens in the reproductive tract. DES is a non-steroidal oestrogen agonist that was among the first synthetic oestrogens to be developed. It was administered to over 2 million women between 1940 and 1970 as treatment for threatened miscarriage. In mice, neonatal exposure to DES produces endometrial cancer in 95% of animals by 18 months of age. In women, prenatal DES exposure leads to structural abnormalities of the reproductive tract (Chapter 27) and to clear cell adenocarcinoma of the vagina and cervix. The carcinogenic action of the DES appears to be mediated in part through activation of the oestrogen receptor. Whether prenatal DES exposure will cause endometrial cancer in humans will be determined as this cohort of women continues to be followed through menopause. The molecular genetic mechanism by which DES lead to clear cell carcinoma and naturally occurring oestrogens to type I endometrial cancer may be similar. Genetic instability of microsatellite sequences has been demonstrated in both of these tumours.

Molecular biology of endometrial cancer

K-*ras* oncogene mutations and microsatellite instability are most common in type I, oestrogen-related tumours. Mutations of the *PT53* tumour suppressor gene and overexpression of the *ERBB2* oncogene are more frequently observed in the type II, non-oestrogen-related tumours.

Endometrial hyperplasia

Endometrial hyperplasia describes a spectrum of changes in the endometrium. These can range from slightly disordered patterns that merely exaggerate the changes seen in the late proliferative stage of the menstrual cycle to irregular, hyperchromatic lesions that are difficult to distinguish from endometrioid adenocarcinoma. Nonetheless, non-invasive endometrial hyperplasia can be divided into two basic types: hyperplasia and atypical hyperplasia. Atypia is characterized by nuclear enlargement, hyperchromasia or irregularities in nuclear shape. Hyperplastic lesions can be further subdivided. Simple hyperplasia describes hyperplastic changes with regular glandular architecture while complex hyperplasia has irregular glandular architecture. Of the four types of endometrial hyperplasias – simple, complex, atypical simple and atypical complex – only atypical complex hyperplasia poses significant risk for progression to invasive carcinoma. The progression from hyperplasia is slow and may take 5 or more years. About 20% of women with complex atypical hyperplasia will develop endometrial adenocarcinoma. Only 1–2% of those with the other hyperplastic lesions will progress.

Endometrial hyperplasia has the same epidemiological risk factors as endometrial cancer. Among patients with atypical endometrial hyperplasia, postmenopausal status is associated with the highest risk of progression to adenocarcinoma (33% over 10 years). Endometrial

cancer is rare during the child-bearing years. When it occurs, it is usually associated with clinical disorders that cause chronic, unopposed oestrogen exposure, including the polycystic ovary syndrome and chronic anovulation (Chapter 31). Oestrogen-producing ovarian tumours, such as the granulosa–theca cell tumours (Chapter 41), are also associated with the development of endometrial hyperplasia and adenocarcinoma in premenopausal women.

Progesterone-based therapies are used to halt endometrial proliferation and to convert the endometrium to a secretory state in women with endometrial hyperplasia with low malignant potential. Treatment can be given cyclically or continuously. Atypical endometrial hyperplasia is treated surgically (hysterectomy) unless there is a contraindication to the procedure.

Incidence of endometrial cancer in different countries for women selected by age.

Country	Incidence per 100 000
USA (Almeda, CA; white population)	45.8
Germany (Saarland)	33.8
New Zealand (Maori)	28.8
Switzerland (Geneva)	23.6
Canada (Alberta)	21.1
USA (Almeda, CA; black population)	19.3
Malta	17.8
Sweden	16.8
Israel	15.0
Finland	13.4
Poland (Warsaw)	13.2
Romania (Timis)	12.4
UK (Liverpool)	12.0
Puerto Rico	8.4
Columbia (Cali)	7.0
Singapore (Cinesi)	6.8
Spain (Saaragozza)	5.8
Brazil (Recife)	3.0
India (Bombay)	1.8
Japan (Miyagi)	1.7

Risk factors for endometrial cancer

Increased risk
Obesity
Diabetes
High fat diet
High socioeconomic status
Urban residence
Positive family history
Polycystic ovary syndrome
Unopposed oestrogen replacement therapy in menopause
Tamoxifen use
Oestrogen-secreting tumours

Decreased risk
Delayed menarche
Combination oral contraceptive use
Child-bearing

Overview

Invasive squamous cell carcinoma accounts for 80% of cervical malignancies. Unlike the remainder of the reproductive tract cancers, which are more prevalent in industrialized countries, cervical cancer is the number one cancer killer among women in the third world. Its epidemiology suggests that it is a sexually transmitted disease. Squamous cancer of the cervix is unique in that it is a preventable disease when proper screening and treatment are available and employed.

Like prostatic cancer in men (Chapter 40), cervical cancer typically arises from a precursor lesion, cervical intraepithelial neoplasia (CIN). CIN is asymptomatic and appears to precede invasive carcinoma of the cervix by 5–15 years. Almost all cervical cancer arises in the transformation zone (squamocolumnar junction) of the cervix. Here, the columnar, glandular epithelium of the endocervix meets the squamous epithelium of the ectocervix. The location of the squamocolumnar junction changes in response to a variety of factors and is different in young postpubertal girls when compared to postmenopausal women (see figure below). In older women, the transformation zone may be high in the endocervical canal. This makes the early diagnosis of cervical neoplasia more difficult in this population.

There are three general types of overt cervical cancers. The most common is characterized by a large friable exophytic lesion that extends into the vagina and bleeds profusely when touched. Other tumours infiltrate the cervical stroma and create 'barrel-shaped' lesions without outward signs of growth. These barrel-shaped lesions can first present when their local spread causes urinary or bowel symptoms. The last group of cervical cancers are ulcerative tumours that often replace the cervix and upper vagina with a large purulent crater.

Cervical carcinomas can spread in any one of four ways: (i) directly into the vaginal mucosa; (ii) directly into the myometrium of the lower uterine segment; (iii) into the paracervical lymphatics and from there to the obturator, hypogastric and external iliac lymph nodes; and (iv) directly into adjacent structures such as the bladder anteriorly, the rectum posteriorly, or into the parametrial tissues and pelvic sidewalls laterally. Lymphatic invasion can occur even when cervical tumours are still small. Haematogenous spread and distant metastases are usually very late manifestations of the disease.

Surgical treatment is used for early stage cervical cancers.

A combination of radiation and chemotherapy is used for patients with advanced disease and in those who are poor surgical candidates.

Epidemiology of cervical cancer

The association of sexual activity with cervical cancer was first identified over 150 years ago when it was noted that the disease was rare in nuns and frequent in prostitutes. Subsequent epidemiological data have identified the onset of sexual activity in adolescence and multiple sexual partners as high-risk characteristics for cervical cancer. Its incidence is higher in low-income women but this effect is not independent of early sexual activity and multiple sex partners. Smoking is an independent risk factor for the development of cervical cancer. Characteristics of a 'high-risk' male partner have been identified; men whose previous partner developed cervical cancer or who themselves develop penile cancer put their sexual partner at increased risk.

Epidemiological data suggesting that cervical cancer behaves like a sexually transmitted disease provoked studies into potential causative agents. Virtually everything that can be found in, or put in, the female genital tract has been implicated as the sexually transmitted agent. The most likely candidate for a causative agent is the human papillomavirus (HPV), although more recent epidemiological data indicate that HPV infection alone is insufficient. While as many as 85% of cervical cancers contain high-risk HPV sequences, the prevalence of HPV infection in control groups without any evidence of cervical neoplasia is much too high for this infection alone to account for the cancers.

Pathogenesis of squamous cell neoplasia of the cervix

Because the cervix is so physically accessible, the pathogenesis of cervical neoplasia has been studied extensively. Pathogenesis clearly involves exposure of a vulnerable tissue (the transformation zone) to carcinogens. Some degree of host compromise is also likely involved.

The squamocolumnar junction is one of six epithelial boundaries present within the lower genital tract. It is discernible from the 24th week of fetal life throughout adulthood. The position of the squamocolumnar junction is affected by the hormonal and anatomical changes of puberty, pregnancy and menopause. Prior to puberty, the squamocolumnar junction usually lies at the position of the external cervical os

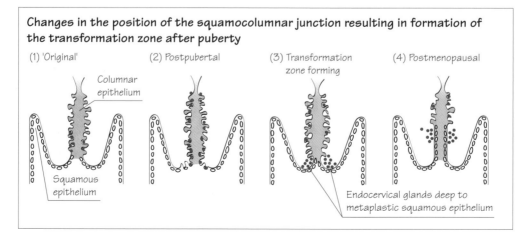

Changes in the position of the squamocolumnar junction resulting in formation of the transformation zone after puberty

(1) 'Original' (2) Postpubertal (3) Transformation zone forming (4) Postmenopausal

Columnar epithelium

Squamous epithelium

Endocervical glands deep to metaplastic squamous epithelium

(Chapter 10). With puberty, oestrogen-induced changes in the shape and volume of the cervix carry the squamocolumnar junction out onto the anatomical ectocervix. This repositioning exposes tissues previously found in the lower endocervical canal to the vagina. The exposure of the simple mucin-secreting epithelium to the acidic vaginal environment induces a chemical denaturation of the villus tips of the columnar epithelium. The reparative process that follows eventually produces a mature squamous epithelium. The first sign of the reparative process is the appearance of activated 'reserve cells' beneath the columnar epithelium. The reserve cells gradually become stratified beneath the columnar cells and replace the columnar cells, forming the transformation zone. **After menopause, the squamocolumnar junction retreats to a position high within the endocervical canal**.

HPV is a DNA virus that causes epithelial lesions in the gastrointestinal tract, skin, cervix and vulva (Chapter 46). Its genetic structure is known and two of its nine genes, *E6* and *E7*, appear to have oncogenic potential. It is these sequences that are found in the nuclei of precursor cervical neoplastic lesions and that are integrated into the host chromosomes in invasive cervical cancer. Integration is associated with de-repression of the *E6* and *E7* genes. This allows them to function as oncogenes. The gene products from *E6* and *E7* interact with the tumour suppressor genes, *RB-1* and *TP53*, and disrupt normal growth regulation of host cells. The *E6* and *E7* genes of HPV can transform cells *in vitro*.

More than 100 types of HPV have been identified to date. Cervical cells with cytological abnormalities and those from cervical cancers most commonly contain sequences from HPV6, HPV11, HPV16 or HPV18. HPV6 and 11 are associated with low risk for malignancy. In distinct contrast, 85% of cervical cancers contain HPV16 or 18 sequences.

Using sensitive molecular techniques, recent epidemiological data have identified a very high prevalence of genital tract exposure to HPV in the general population and a discrepancy in the previous pathogenetic hypotheses. Many women infected with HPV do not develop cervical neoplasic changes. Numerous investigators have attempted to reconcile the epidemiology of HPV infection with its known oncogenic effects *in vitro*. It is now thought that the immune response of the host may play a key role in whether HPV exposure leads to cervical neoplasia. Supporting this hypothesis is the extremely high incidence of cervical neoplasia seen among patients with immune deficiencies, including women infected with the HIV virus and women taking immunosuppressive medications following kidney transplants. CIN rates in HIV-positive women are 10 times higher than controls, and transplant patients have rates approaching 40%.

Cervical intraepithelial neoplasia (CIN) is the term used to encompass all epithelial abnormalities of the cervix. It has replaced an older terminology that used the terms 'dysplasia' and 'carcinoma *in situ*' of the cervix. **CIN, although divided into grades, is actually a single neoplastic continuum**. The designations CIN I, II and III reflect the extent of the cellular aberrations within the cervical epithelium. In CIN I, the lower one-third of the epithelial cells lack evidence of cytoplasmic differentiation or maturation. In CIN II, the changes of CIN I occupy two-thirds of the epithelium. In CIN III, these changes are present throughout the full thickness of the epithelium.

The diagnosis of CIN is made on biopsy specimens taken as part of the evaluation for an abnormal Pap smear screen. Treatment is dependent on the severity of the abnormalities seen in the specimen and other clinical variables.

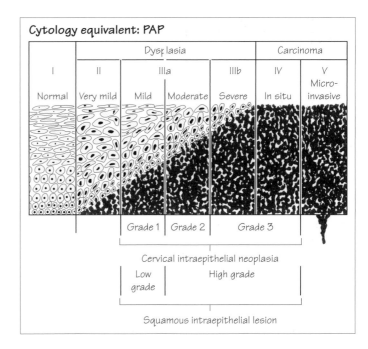

Pap smear screening for cervical neoplasia

The cervical smear or Pap test (named after Dr George Papanicolaou who developed the test) was designed as a screening test to detect squamous cell abnormalities. Its success is based on the fact that the nuclear abnormalities of dysplastic cervical cells are present in samples that are scraped or exfoliated from the surface of the cervix. Pap smears can also detect cancer, but the detection of a cancer is actually considered a failure of the screening programme, which is designed to identify and permit treatment of intraepithelial lesions before they progress to cancer.

Adequate Pap smear screening can reduce a woman's chance of dying from cervical cancer by 90%. Currently it is recommended that all women who are sexually active or have reached the age of 18 have an annual Pap smear screening and pelvic exam. Once three satisfactory normal exams and Pap smears have been obtained, the interval may be increased at the discretion of the woman's physician. New diagnosis and treatment algorithms include the use of reflexive HPV testing in conjunction with cervical cytology. This approach appears to be particularly useful when cytological testing discovers abnormalities of otherwise undetermined significance. The presence of high-risk HPV subtypes in these patients indicate more aggressive diagnostic and therapeutic interventions.

Cervical adenocarcinoma

Adenocarcinoma of the cervix is much rarer than squamous cell lesions. It occurs most often in women during the reproductive years. Although adenocarcinoma *in situ* is thought to be the precursor lesion of invasive cervical adenocarcinoma, the timing of progression from precursor to invasion is not known. Cervical cytology does not reliably detect adenocarcinomas. These lesions do not appear to be associated with HPV infection, although cervical squamous neoplasia is concomitantly present in 30–50% of cervical adenocarcinomas.

Imprinting

Imprinting is the differential expression of a gene or set of genes that is determined by whether that genetic material was inherited from the mother or from the father. During the imprinting process, specific genes are methylated so that they can no longer be transcribed. Therefore, for certain genetic loci, only the information from one parent is transcriptionally active. When a gene is maternally imprinted, the gene acquired from the mother is inactive and that from the father is transcribed. With paternal imprinting, the allele acquired from the father is inactive. Normal embryonic development requires that one set of genes be maternally imprinted and a second paternally imprinted. Therefore, a zygote must not only have a $2n$ chromosome content but each of the $1n$ components must derive from different parents. Several tumours of the reproductive system have helped us to better understand the process of imprinting and the consequences of imprinting abnormalities.

Gestational trophoblastic disease (GTD), dermoid cysts of the ovary, and germ-cell tumours (GCTs) of the testis all display abnormalities in imprinting. GTD and dermoid tumours contain two sets of chromosomes from a single parent, so there exists no opportunity for biparental imprinting. Two sets of maternally imprinted genes are present in dermoid tumours of the ovary. The result is development of disorganized fetal tissues without any supporting placenta or fetal membranes. Conversely, two sets of paternally imprinted genes are present in GTD. In these cases, dysplastic trophoblast develops, but a fetus does not. GCTs of the testis have taught different lessons concerning the importance of imprinting. GCTs that arise in immature and incompletely imprinted cells are more aggressive than those that arise in fully imprinted germ cells.

Gestational trophoblastic disease

Gestational trophoblastic disease (GTD) is one of the earliest reported neoplasms. Hippocrates first described 'dropsy' of the uterus in 400 BC and a 13th-century tombstone noted the birth of 365 'children', half boys and half girls, to the woman buried there. Today GTD, also called molar pregnancy, retains its leading position in tumour biology as the most sensitive and curable of all human cancers. The genetic origin of molar pregnancies has also played a pivotal part in our understanding of the role of the maternal and paternal genome in embryonic development.

There are a spectrum of diseases within the GTD classification: hydatidiform mole, either complete (CHM) or partial (PHM), persistent, non-metastatic GTD, metastatic good-prognosis GTD and metastatic poor-prognosis GTD. The latter includes aggressive tumours known as choriocarcinomas (CC). Of these, CHM and PHM follow abnormal conceptions and are restricted to women. Choriocarcinoma is unique among GTD in that it can arise from a normal conception, a molar pregnancy or a germ-cell line. Choriocarcinoma in men is exclusively of germ-cell origin (Chapter 39).

CHM and PHM contain two sets of paternal chromosomes. The former has only paternally derived genomic DNA. This situation promotes the development of placental tissues in the absence of fetal tissue development. In PHM, two sets of paternal chromosomes are accompanied by a single set of maternal chromosomes. Again, the paternally imprinted genes are duplicated and placental overgrowth occurs. Here, maternally imprinted genes are also present and fetal tissue development is seen.

Complete hydatidiform mole

CHM is the most common of the GTDs and occurs in about 1/1000–1/1500 pregnancies in Western countries. It is at least twice as common in Asia and less common in black races. Extremes of age increase the risk for CHM, with women under 15 and over 40 at highest risk. Other risk factors include previous history of CHM, previous miscarriage, maternal balanced chromosomal translocation, professional occupation and perhaps deficiencies in animal fat and carotene in the diet. A previously normal pregnancy lowers the risk of CHM.

CHM is characterized histologically by the presence of large amounts of hydropic placental villi and no fetal tissue. It presents clinically with delayed menses and the diagnosis of pregnancy. Pregnancy symptoms such as nausea and vomiting are often exaggerated because of the high human chorionic gonadotropin (hCG) production by the abnormal trophoblast. Some patients with CHM will be hyperthyroid because hCG exhibits some intrinsic thyroid-stimulating activity.

Women with CHM who want to preserve their fertility are treated by removing the molar tissue from the uterine cavity (uterine evacuation). Those who do not desire future fertility may choose hysterectomy. Eighty per cent of CHMs will respond to these approaches. Those who have persistent disease require chemotherapy and the vast majority will

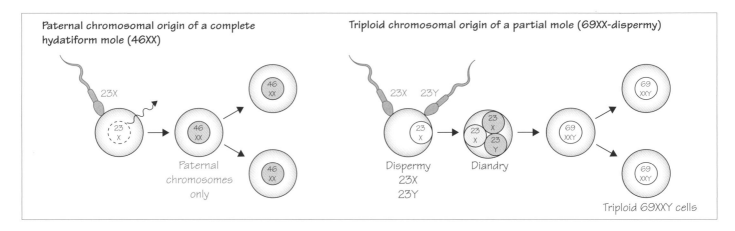

Paternal chromosomal origin of a complete hydatiform mole (46XX)

Triploid chromosomal origin of a partial mole (69XX-dispermy)

ultimately be cured. CHM is exquisitely sensitive to antimetabolite chemotherapy, typically methotrexate with folate rescue.

The unique genetic origins of CHM were suspected well before the advent of modern molecular techniques when karyotype analyses revealed that 96% of them were 46XX. Polymerase chain reaction and restriction fragment length polymorphism (RFLP) analyses have demonstrated that **while CHM is always diploid, the chromosomes are all of paternal origin**. Most CHMs arise from fertilization of an enucleate, or empty egg, with a single 23X sperm. This paternal haplotype reduplicates and the 46XX karyotype results. The remaining CHMs arise after fertilization of the enucleate egg with two sperm (dispermy); of these about one-quarter (4% of the total CHMs) will have a 46XY karyotype. All CHM have maternal mitochondrial DNA and this confirms that the oocyte cell machinery is involved. To date, the mechanism by which the egg enucleates is not known. Some hypothesize that the maternal chromosomes degenerate, others pose that the female pronucleus is extruded with the polar body.

Partial hydatidiform mole
PHM exists when proliferative villi with hydropic degeneration coexist with a fetus. The fetus is genetically abnormal and will commonly die by the late first or early second trimester. The villous hydropic changes seen in PHM are not as pronounced as those in CHM and may be missed on ultrasonographic examination. Pathological examination of the placenta is often necessary to make the diagnosis. Patients with PHM tend to be older than those with CHM. PHM has a lower risk of subsequent malignancy than does CHM.

PHM pregnancies are all triploid and contain two copies of the paternal genome. PHM pregnancies most commonly arise from dispermic fertilization (diandry). They occasionally occur after fertilization by a diploid sperm that failed to undergo a first or second reduction division during meiosis.

Persistent and metastatic gestational trophoblastic disease
Persistent and metastatic GTD are typically preceded by CHM. They occasionally follow PHM or even normal pregnancies. Persistent GTD can invade the uterus or metastasize to liver, lung and brain. Even metastatic disease has a very high cure rate with appropriate treatment.

Genetic study of neoplastic trophoblastic tissue is very important to the patient because gestational tumours have a better than 90% cure rate whereas non-gestational tumours with trophoblastic differentiation are essentially lethal.

Dermoid tumours
Benign ovarian teratomas, also known as **dermoids**, arise from 'parthenogenetic' activation of premeiotic oocytes. Parthenogenetic activation of the oocyte stimulates oocyte mitosis in the absence of the male pronucleus and its accompanying DNA. Parthenogenetic activation can be induced *in vitro* by a variety of methods, including chemical and electrical exposure. The stimuli that drive parthenogenesis in the formation of ovarian teratomas are not known. All the chromosomes in an ovarian dermoid tumour are maternally derived and, therefore, maternally imprinted. The tumours are characterized by disorganized overgrowth of many of the cell types normally seen in fetuses. This includes hair, bone, cartilage, adipose tissue and glandular derivatives (Chapter 41). Not surprisingly, trophoblast-derived tissue is seldom present.

Ovarian dermoid tumours arise from more mature germ cells than the other female GCTs. Like other GCTs, the molecular event(s) that lead to activation of the germ cells can occur *in utero*, and indeed dermoid tumours have been detected in the fetus and newborn.

GCTs of the testis
Spermatocytic seminomas are unique among the GCTs of the testis in that they are found in older men and are typically slow-growing (Chapter 39). This less aggressive behaviour may occur because spermatocytic seminomas arise from mature spermatogonia rather than spermatogonial stem cells. During the development of spermatazoa, the diploid (biparental) spermatogonial stem cell must undergo reduction division to the haploid state. It is equally important that the DNA in these haploid cells be completely uniparental. If this occurs, appropriate paternally imprinted DNA will be transmitted during fertilization. Imprinting appears to occur during spermatocyte maturation some time after the second meiotic division halves the chromosome number. When neoplastic transformation occurs in immature testicular germ cells, the biparental imprinting of the cells preserves pluripotentiality and allows the development of less differentiated, aggressive tumours with embryonal or trophoblastic components. When transformation occurs in more mature and fully imprinted spermatogonium, the tumours are less aggressive (spermatocytic seminomas).

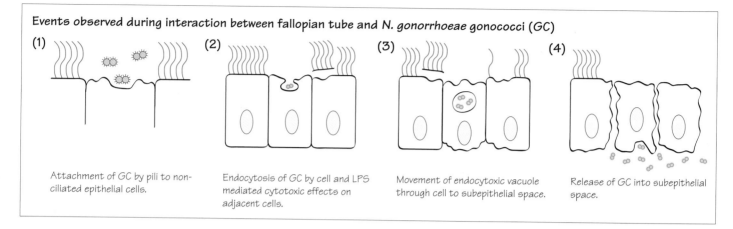

Events observed during interaction between fallopian tube and *N. gonorrhoeae* gonococci (GC)

(1) Attachment of GC by pili to non-ciliated epithelial cells.

(2) Endocytosis of GC by cell and LPS mediated cytotoxic effects on adjacent cells.

(3) Movement of endocytoxic vacuole through cell to subepithelial space.

(4) Release of GC into subepithelial space.

Gonorrhoea

Overview

Gonorrhoea is the most frequently reported communicable disease in many more-developed countries. Rates are 5–50 times higher than in the less-developed world. The Gram-negative coccus that causes the disease is called **Neisseria gonorrhoeae**. It is a highly specialized organism that requires a mucosal surface to gain access to the body. **The most important health consequence of gonorrhoeal infections is Fallopian tube damage and the associated predisposition to ectopic (tubal) pregnancies and infertility**.

In men, urethritis is the most common clinical manifestation of gonorrhoea. Symptoms include dysuria and/or a purulent urethral discharge. Local complications of gonorrhoea are uncommon in men, although urethral stricture, epididymitis and prostatitis can occur. Between 20 and 30% of heterosexual men with symptomatic gonococcal urethritis are simultaneously infected with *Chlamydia trachomatis*.

Gonococcal infection in women is often asymptomatic. Morbidity associated with the infection, however, is far greater than that seen among infected men. Ironically, a significant number of women diagnosed with gonorrhoea are identified in sexually transmitted disease (STD) clinics as the asymptomatic consort of an infected partner. Uncomplicated urogenital gonococcal infection in women may present as dysuria from urethritis, vaginal discharge from cervicitis or purulent drainage from the Skene's or Bartholin's glands at the vaginal introitus. **Pelvic inflammatory disease (PID)** is a term used to describe infection of the upper genital tract and includes endometritis, salpingitis and peritonitis. *Neisseria gonorrhoeae* and *C. trachomatis* are the two pathogens most frequently isolated from women with positive cultures for PID. Women with gonococcal PID present with lower abdominal pain, abnormal uterine bleeding, dyspareunia (pain on intercourse) and fever. Although mortality from PID is low, morbidity is extremely high. PID is an important risk factor for chronic pelvic pain, infertility and tubal pregnancies. In some areas of Africa, up to 50% of women are infertile as a result of tubal occlusion from gonococcal PID.

Other serious clinical manifestations include disseminated gonococcal infection (DGI) and gonococcal ophthalmia neonatorum, a severe form of conjunctivitis affecting newborns who acquire the infection in the birth canal. Neonatal gonococcal ophthalmia can result in blindness if left untreated. It is a rarity in developed countries because occular prophylaxis is mandated at birth, but remains a significant problem in many parts of the underdeveloped world.

Gonorrhoea is treated with antibiotics. The choice of antibiotic continues to evolve because of the propensity for the organism to be associated with other STDs and to develop antibiotic resistance.

Epidemiology of gonorrhoea

Gonorrhoea is largely a disease of youth. Incidence peaks in men and women at ages 18–24 years. In addition to age, the risk factors include low socioeconomic status, urban residence, unmarried status, non-white race, male homosexuality and prostitution.

Biology of *N. gonorrhoeae*

Gonococci enter the body by attaching to non-ciliated columnar mucosal epithelial cells using specialized surface structures on the bacteria known as **pili**. Following attachment by the pili, the gonococci are endocytosed by the cell. At this stage, a lipopolysaccharide (LPS; endotoxin)-mediated event is activated and nearby cells are killed. Following endocytosis of the bacteria, vacuoles containing viable and replicating gonococci pass through the cell from the mucosal surface to the subepithelial membrane. Here, they are released into the underlying tissues. The surface damage caused by the gonococcus allows other pathogens, such as chlamydia, to gain access to the upper reproductive tract and cause multiorganism PID. Movement of the gonococci to subepithelial sites also explains the frequent failure to document its presence in the Fallopian tube despite cervical culture-positive PID.

Gonococci develop their antibiotic resistance through plasmid-mediated and chromosomal mechanisms. Most plasmid-mediated resistance is to penicillin and tetracycline. Chromosomally mediated resistance is more general and involves mutations that alter cell wall permeability or the affinity of binding proteins to antibiotics.

Chlamydia

Overview

There are many similarities between the infections caused by *N. gonorrhoeae* and **Chlamydia trachomatis (CT)**. Chlamydiae gain access to the body by invading the same epithelial cells of the endocervix, urethra, endometrium, Fallopian tubes, rectum and conjunctivae that are host to the gonococcus. Infections in men are relatively asymptomatic and of low morbidity; the major consequence of infection in the male is the risk of transmission to a female partner. In women, gonococcal and chlamydial infections can result in PID, chronic pain, infertility and ectopic pregnancy. There is risk to the newborn from a birth canal infected with gonococci or chlamydiae. The greatest clinical difference between female infection with GC and CT is that **chlamydial PID is often asymptomatic. Hence, chlamydial infection is a major public health hazard because of the potential for unrecognized serious damage to the upper reproductive tracts of women.**

Chlamydia trachomatis is *the* most common STD in the USA and Europe. Chlamydiae are unique bacteria. Like viruses, they are obligate intracellular parasites and can only be propagated in cell culture. Chlamydia causes about 50% of the cases of non-gonococcal urethritis in men. In women, chlamydia can cause mucopurulent cervicitis and the 'urethral syndrome'. In the latter, pain on urination is associated with the presence of white blood cells, but no bacteria, in the urine. Unlike gonorrhoea, chlamydial infection of the upper genital tract often invades the endometrium without causing overt signs of PID. Such subclinical infection may first be recognized with diagnosis of the consequent infertility or ectopic pregnancy.

Several strains of chlamydia cause a unique disorder known as **lymphogranuloma venereum (LGV)**, a chronic disease that, like syphilis, has three clinical stages. The primary lesion of LGV is a small, inconspicuous papule of the genitalia that quickly and quietly disappears. The secondary stage of LGV is characterized by fever, malaise and either acute lymphadenitis of the inguinal region (bubo formation = inguinal syndrome) and/or acute haemorrhagic proctitis (anogenitorectal syndrome). Most people recover uneventfully from the second stage. In an unfortunate few, the chlamydiae persist in the anogenital tissues and incite a chronic inflammatory response that can cause genital tract ulcers, fistulae and strictures. LGV is endemic in much of the less-developed world but sporadic in the USA and Europe. Neonates exposed to chlamydia in the birth canal may develop afebrile pneumonia or conjunctivitis that can progress to blindness.

Unlike gonococci, chlamydiae require prolonged treatment to eradicate the intracellular reservoir of the bacteria. Because of the frequent coexistence of gonorrhoea and chlamydial infection, most treatment regimens include one antibiotic to treat the gonococci and another to treat the chlamydia. True antibiotic resistance is rare in chlamydial infections.

Epidemiology of chlamydial infection

Chlamydia infection is a disease of the young. Additional risk factors include low socioeconomic status, a high number of sexual partners and oral contraceptive use. Barrier methods of contraception (condom, diaphragm, diaphragm plus spermicide) reduce risk.

Biology of chlamydia

The chlamydiae are structurally complex microorganisms. Like viruses, chlamydiae are obligate intracellular parasites. They are classified as bacteria because they contain both DNA and RNA. Like Gram-negative bacteria, they possess outer membrane proteins and a lipopolysaccharide (LPS). Chlamydiae differ from all other bacteria in that their growth cycle is characterized by transformation between two distinct forms: the **elementary body** and the **reticulate body**. The elementary body is a highly infectious, rigid extracellular growth form that is metabolically inactive. The elementary body attaches to non-ciliated columnar or cuboidal epithelial cells and induces ingestion by the host cell. The elementary body-containing phagosome does not fuse with host cell lysosomes, a characteristic crucial to CT survival and unique to only a few organisms (*Mycobacterium tuberculosis* is another). Within the phagosome, the elementary body reorganizes into a larger, metabolically active, fragile and non-infectious reticulate body. The reticulate bodies divide repeatedly by binary fission within the phagosome of the host cell. They will ultimately reorganize back into infectious elementary bodies that are released when the host cell dies.

There are 15 different serotypes or serovars of chlamydiae. These serovars are identified as A through K, Ba, and L_1, L_2 and L_3. Strains D–K are associated with chlamydial STDs. L_1, L_2 and L_3 cause LGV.

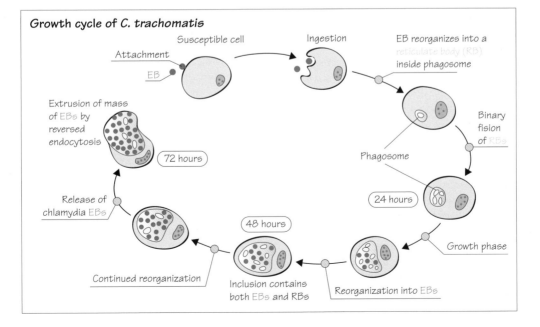

Growth cycle of C. trachomatis

Sexually transmitted diseases of viral origin

Genital warts

Overview

Genital warts are one of the most common diagnoses among patients attending sexually transmitted disease (STD) clinics. The infectious agent responsible is the **human papillomavirus (HPV)**, a pathogen that causes a wide variety of clinical diseases. The **association of HPV with genital tract cancers** has brought attention to the typically benign, albeit inconvenient genital wart. The broad spectrum of genital HPV infection includes (i) latent infection; (ii) subclinical infection; (iii) clinically apparent lesion (condylomata accuminata, warts); and (iv) HPV-associated neoplasia.

Latent infections are identified by the presence of HPV DNA in tissue samples acquired for epidemiological study. In the absence of tissue collection, latent infections would go unrecognized because neither microscopic nor visible lesions are present. Subclinical infections are subtle, flat lesions seen during colposcopic examination (microscopic magnification *in situ*) of acetic acid-treated tissues. Overt genital warts, also known as condyloma acuminata, are flesh-coloured, pink or pigmented papules with a frond-like surface. Sessile warts, or flat condyloma-like lesions, are less common, accounting for only 20% of visible genital warts. Most genital warts in men are on the penis. In women, they are found most often at the vaginal introitus and on the labia. They less commonly affect the vagina or cervix. Most genital warts are asymptomatic. When symptoms do occur, they are often secondary to local friction-induced irritation from clothing or intercourse. HPV-associated neoplasias include intraepithelial lesions of the cervix (CIN/SIL) and vulva (VIN) and invasive carcinomas at both sites. The role of HPV in cervical neoplasia is reviewed in Chapter 43.

Because most genital warts are sexually transmitted, their presence indicates risk for other STDs. Patients with genital warts should be screened for syphilis, gonorrhoea, chlamydia, hepatitis and human immunodeficiency virus (HIV). Treatment of genital warts is locally administered. Destructive therapies use liquid nitrogen or local application of acetic acid. Interestingly, destruction of only a subset of lesions can lead to resolution of untreated lesions. Other therapies include direct application of podyphyllin, a naturally occurring resin that poisons the mitotic spindle and arrests viral propagation. Immune-based approaches use local application of imiquimod, an immune modulator that induces local production of inflammatory cytokines and T-cell mediated cytolysis of virally infected cells. Treatments aim to remove symptomatic warts. None are effective in eradicating the virus.

Epidemiology of genital warts

Most genital warts are seen in young people, aged 16–25 years. Because most infections are subclinical and unrecognized, epidemiological data on symptomatic infections are certainly biased. Cross-sectional studies on the prevalence of HPV DNA in cervical cytological specimens have shown that 15–25% of women aged 20–25 years are HPV positive; about 5% are positive for high-risk HPV subtypes (e.g. HPV type 16). By age 35 years, the overall prevalence has decreased to 5% and only 1% of screened women are positive for subtype HPV16. Penile swabs are positive for HPV DNA in about 5% of men.

Most HPV infections are acquired sexually. Approximately 60% of the sexual partners of patients with genital warts will themselves develop genital warts. The average incubation time is 2–3 months. Infectivity appears to decrease over time. Although rare, it is possible to acquire HPV through non-sexual transmission. Neonates can become infected during delivery.

Molecular biology of human papillomaviruses

HPV is a member of the Papovaviridae family of DNA viruses. Other well-known members of this family are the polyomaviruses (polio virus and SV40). The virology of HPV has been difficult to study because it is rarely isolated in its viable free form and it cannot be propagated in cell culture. Virus-containing material is available only from excised warts. In cutaneous warts, the viral genome is a double-stranded circular DNA molecule. In most HPV-associated lesions, the viral DNA is present as an extrachromosomal episome. In some cancers, viral DNA is integrated into the host chromosomal DNA.

Of the 70 different HPV genotypes identified, only types 6, 11, 16, 18, 31, 33 and 35 are associated with genital lesions. Types 6 and 11 are most commonly identified in genital warts, and types 16 and 18 with neoplasia (high-risk subtypes). HPV subtypes 1–5 are associated with common skin warts and plantar warts.

The papillomavirus genome has been extensively analysed. It includes only nine genes. Genes *E1* and *E2* are the sites of integration into host DNA. Genes *E1* and *E2* function as repressors of genes *E6* and *E7* in the intact virus. When host integration occurs, *E1* and *E2* are disrupted and *E6* and *E7* are overexpressed. *E6* and *E7* are capable of interfering with important tumour suppressor proteins in the host cell. Their overexpression is associated with neoplastic transformation, explaining the oncogenic potential of HPV.

Genital herpes

Overview

Genital herpes is an STD that doesn't go away. Instead, the responsible agent, **herpes simplex virus (HSV)**, establishes a latent infection

Human papillomavirus genes

*E1**	Necessary for viral DNA replication
	May have a role as repressor of immortalization
*E2**	Necessary for viral DNA replication along with *E1*
E3	?
E4	Intracellular protein that interacts with cytokeratin
	? Confers tissue specificity on HPV type
E5	Activates platelet-derived growth factor (PDGF) receptor in host
	Transforms proliferative signal to the cell
E6[†]	Interacts with p53, a tumour suppressor product monitoring DNA damage
	Transforming signal
E7[†]	Interacts with Rb-1, the retinoblastoma gene, a tumour suppressor gene that gates the cell cycle
	Strong, transforming signal
L1	Major capsid protein
L2	Minor capsid protein

* Mutations in *E1* and/or *E2* result in integration of viral DNA into host DNA.

[†] Disruption of growth regulation necessary to propagate virus.

in the sacral dorsal root ganglia. It can be reactivated from latency by a variety of circumstances, including fever, sun exposure, and hormonal changes. Herpetic infection causes the greatest morbidity in the neonate, who acquires it from the genital tract of the mother at delivery, and in immunocompromised patients for whom its disseminated form can be life-threatening. Genital HSV infection has been linked with risk for cervical cancer, suggesting that it may act with HPV as a cofactor in neoplastic transformation or may promote HPV transmission.

There are two distinct serological types of HSV: HSV-1 and HSV-2. HSV-1 infection is typically asymptomatic and almost ubiquitous. It is transmitted by primary infection of the respiratory tract. HSV-1 has been found in the trigeminal ganglion of 80% of cadavers. While HSV-1 reactivation typically causes 'cold sores' or 'fever blisters', primary infection or reinfection with a new strain can cause encephalitis and blinding keratoconjunctivitis.

HSV-2 has a predilection for genital disease, although HSV-1 infections of the genitalia and HSV-2 infections of the oral cavity do occur. HSV-2 is much more likely than HSV-1 to become a latent infection of the sacral ganglion and to cause neonatal disease.

Patients with herpetic infections present with three clinical scenarios: **primary first episode**, **non-primary first episode** and **recurrent episodes**. These presentations inform our understanding of the biology and epidemiology of genital HSV infections. First episodes describe the initial recognition by the patient or health-care provider that a genital herpes infection is occurring. In primary first episodes, no HSV antibodies can be detected in acute phase serum samples, demonstrating that there has been no prior HSV infection. HSV antibodies will be present at the time of the first recognized genital herpes outbreak in non-primary first episodes. Recurrent episodes require recognition that the patient has had a prior episode(s) of symptomatic HSV. The severity of clinical manifestations and the incidence of complications at presentation vary according to whether the infection is primary, non-primary or recurrent.

Primary genital HSV disease is typically the most severe, although it is clear that primary infection can also be totally asymptomatic. Over 80% of patients with primary genital HSV will have local painful penile or vulvar lesions, dysuria, urethral or vaginal discharge and painful inguinal adenopathy. Fever, headache, malaise and myalgias are reported in 40% of men and 70% of women. Urinary retention and proctitis can occur from involvement of the autonomic nerves of the bladder and rectum. Aseptic meningitis occurs in 12–30% of patients with primary infections. The mean duration of viral shedding from mucocutaneous lesions in primary genital HSV-2 infections is 2–3 weeks. Non-primary first infections tend to be milder than primary first infections, presumably because acquired humoral and cellular immunity partially contain infectious spread.

Recurrent genital HSV-2 disease typically involves painful recrudescence of the mucocutaneous lesions on the penis or vulva and cervix. Local viral shedding occurs at the site of lesions, although cervical shedding has also been documented in the absence of visible cervical lesions. Systemic symptoms are absent. The mean duration of symptoms and viral shedding is much shorter with recurrences.

Medications that inhibit viral DNA synthesis have been developed to treat the symptoms of HSV infection. Treatment will stop viral DNA replication and spread but will neither prevent latent infections nor eradicate the virus.

Abstinence from sexual contact with an infected partner when lesions are visible is the only way to prevent genital HSV infection.

Unfortunately, even this is not completely protective because transmission can occur during asymptomatic viral shedding. Condoms are also not completely protective. The penile shaft may be partially exposed to the vulva during intercourse using a condom. In addition, the HSV virus is capable of penetrating latex.

Epidemiology of genital HSV infection

Symptomatic genital HSV infection accounts for 2–4% of visits to STD clinics in the UK and the USA. Genital HSV infections are reported more commonly among Caucasians than non-Caucasians. A higher prevalence of anti-HSV-antibodies is noted with decreasing age at first coitus and with increasing number of sexual partners.

The incidence of neonatal herpes is about 1/7500 live births.

Biology of HSV virus

HSV is a member of the herpesvirus class of DNA viruses. Herpesviridae includes two serotypes of HSV (HSV-1 and HSV-2), cytomegalovirus (CMV), varicella zoster (chickenpox, shingles) and Epstein–Barr virus (mononucleosis, chronic fatigue syndrome). Herpesviruses would be better called 'complex' rather than 'simplex' because they have the most complicated structure and replication cycles of all the viruses.

Genital HSV is acquired by sexual contact with contaminated secretions or lesions. Herpesviruses are very susceptible to desiccation and extremes of temperature, making transmission by fomites very rare. Once the virus has gained access to mucosal cells, it destroys the host DNA during productive replication of its own and kills the cell. HSV spreads by contiguity to adjacent cells and tracks toward autonomic nerve endings. Mucosal and skin cells infected with HSV produce serous transudates that result in the classic vesicles seen in the disorder.

Following primary genital mucocutaneous infection, HSV virions travel to the dorsal root ganglia of the sacral plexus (S_2–S_4) via the intra-axonal route. Here, they persist in a non-replicative state until reactivation. Reactivation is heralded by a dramatic increase in viral DNA synthesis. This is followed by spread of virus back down the sensory neurones to the skin. There are currently two theories of reactivation. In the first, stimuli such as physical injury, heat, hormonal perturbations or immunological changes disturb the host ganglion cells. In response, the resident virions renew DNA synthesis and viral replication. In the second theory, small amounts of virus are continually produced by host ganglion cells. These pathogens are in constant transit down the sensory axons to the skin. According to this hypothesis, it is the local conditions that determine when a recurrence will occur.

HSV in pregnancy and the neonate

Ninety per cent of women with primary genital HSV-2 infection shed virus from their cervix during the acute infection. This level drops to 70% in women with primary genital HSV-1 infection and 70% in women with non-primary first episodes of genital HSV-2 infection. These numbers stand in stark contrast to the 12–20% rate of cervical shedding among women with recurrent external genital lesions. It is not surprising; therefore, that 50% of pregnant women with primary genital HSV will transmit infection to the neonate while only 5% of women with recurrent genital HSV will do so. Neonatal herpetic infections are life-threatening. They may be prevented with appropriate use of caesarean delivery.

Syphilis

Natural history of untreated syphilis

Syphilis is caused by a spirochaete, **Treponema pallidum**, which enters the body through miniscule breaks in the skin of the external genitalia that occur during sexual intercourse. Once the spirochaete has entered, the untreated disease progresses through **four consecutive stages: primary, secondary, latent and tertiary syphilis**. Antibiotic treatment at any stage short of tertiary can prevent the late, life-threatening sequelae of the disease. Syphilis may also be transmitted from a woman to her fetus at any point during pregnancy, with serious consequences.

The primary lesion of syphilis, the **chancre**, develops in venereal locations close to where *T. pallidum* typically enters the body: the penis, labia, perineum, anus or rectum. Chancres are painless, small papules that persist for 1–2 months and heal spontaneously.

The secondary stage of syphilis is a disseminated form. Blood-borne spirochaetes populate the dermis throughout the body causing a widespread papular rash over the trunk and extremities. Because the disease is systemic, fever, myalgias, lymphadenopathy, sore throat and headache are common. Secondary syphilis can also be associated with immune complex deposition in the joints, kidneys and eyes, leading to arthritis, glomerulonephritis, nephrotic syndrome and uveitis. Untreated secondary syphilis resolves over 4–12 weeks, leaving the patient symptom free. The subsequent months to years until the onset of symptoms of tertiary syphilis is known as the latent period.

Tertiary syphilis usually appears many years after the disseminated stage. Tertiary syphilis can involve multiple organs, including the cardiovascular and nervous systems. Overall, about one-quarter of untreated patients develop recognizable late (tertiary) complications of syphilis, one-quarter have asymptomatic lesions demonstrable at autopsy and half have no anatomical lesions attributable to syphilis present at autopsy. About half of the patients with symptomatic tertiary syphilis will die as a direct result of the disease, typically of cardiovascular complications.

Infection of the placenta and fetus will occur in virtually 100% of pregnant women who suffer the spirochaetemia accompanying primary or secondary syphilis. Complications of syphilis in pregnancy include miscarriage, stillbirth, premature delivery and congenital syphilis. The manifestations of congenital syphilis are protean. Its neonatal mortality rate is 50%.

Syphilis is treated with penicillin in all but highly allergic patients.

Epidemiology of syphilis

Syphilis was very common in many parts of the world until antibiotic therapy became available in the 1940s. The prevalence of the disease fell dramatically after World War II but began to increase again in the 1960s. Up to 75% of cases go unreported. Women and men at high risk for contracting syphilis are young, from lower socioeconomic groups, and have multiple sexual partners. Some 10–50 syphilitic organisms are sufficient to cause infection and about one-third of the sexual contacts of an infected person will become infected. The incidence of congenital syphilis parallels that in women and is increasing. Mandatory prenatal screening has reduced the incidence of late congenital syphilis; late or absent prenatal care is the biggest risk factor for congenital syphilis.

Biology of *T. pallidum*

Treponema pallidum is a member of the bacterial order *Spirochaetaceae*, and closely related to two other treponemas responsible for human disease: *Treponema pertenue*, which causes yaws and *T. carateum*, which causes pinta. Neither electron microscopic examination nor DNA analyses can distinguish between these three organisms. It is believed that the different diseases that develop reflect adaptations of the organism and the host to different points of entry into the body.

Treponema pallidum is a relatively fragile organism that cannot survive for more than a few hours outside moist areas of the body. Its microbiology is very poorly understood because the organism cannot be maintained in cell culture.

Most of the manifestations of syphilis are secondary to the inflammatory reaction caused by the organism. Polymorphonuclear cells (PMNs) arriving at the site of the inoculum ingest the spirochaetes but do not kill them. Lymphocytes and macrophages are recruited to the site. They also surround, but do not kill the treponemes. Antitreponemal antibodies are produced, sometimes in quantities that cause immune complex glomerulonephritis. It remains both amazing and unknown how *T. pallidum* is able to evade host defences and establish an infection. The site of primary infection is surrounded by a mucoid material composed of hyaluronic acid and chondroitin sulphate that may alter the host defences. The best clue available to explain the persistence of disease is the finding that delayed type sensitivity to treponemal antigens is absent in secondary syphilis. New spirochaetes inoculated into the system are not infectious while the original infection persists. This is a common mechanism in chronic parasitic diseases, called 'premunition'; the host resists reinfection but cannot clear the initial infection.

Once the systemic phase of the infection is established, spirochaetes are present virtually everywhere in the infected tissues. Inflammation, however, occurs preferentially around small vessels and causes intimal hyperplasia and obliterative endarteritis. The subsequent focal ischaemic necrosis and fibrosis is responsible for the many late manifestations of the disease.

The inflammatory changes caused by the spirochaetes are most striking in congenital syphilis. The placenta is diffusely fibrotic with inflammation and necrosis of the fetal blood vessels in the placental villi. The resulting vascular insufficiency leads to poor fetal growth (**intrauterine growth restriction**) and **stillbirth**. Fibrosis of the liver and spleen cause fetal anaemia. Compensatory extramedullary haematopoeisis promotes hepatosplenomegaly and the development of pleural effusions and ascites (**fetal hydrops**). Some infants will have a skin rash that closely resembles that of secondary syphilis. A runny nasal discharge loaded with spirochaetes (**snuffles**) may be the only hint of congenital syphilis at birth.

The late manifestations of syphilis, both congenital and tertiary, involve vasculitis and parenchymal damage in the central nervous system.

Human immunodeficiency virus (HIV)

Natural history of untreated HIV infections

The first description of human disease associated with HIV infection surfaced in the early 1980s. Acute infection was reported to cause a 'mononucleosis-like syndrome' with fever, malaise, muscle aches, headache, fatigue, generalized rash, sore throat, lymphadenopathy and

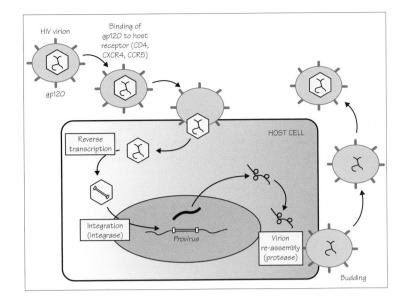

characteristic mucocutaneous lesions. The rapidity of symptom onset after initial contact may reflect the route of viral entry and the viral load of the exposure. Symptoms of primary infection often persist for 2–3 weeks before resolving spontaneously. The disease then enters an asymptomatic phase. This can last from several months to many years. The length of this symptom-free phase appears to depend on the pathogenicity of the infecting viral strain. Co-infection with other viruses or other sexually transmitted disease (STD) pathogens may speed disease progression. During the asymptomatic phase, viral replication continues within infected lymphoid cells (mainly CD4+ T cells). Infected immune cells are destroyed by the virus and, eventually, the host becomes immunocompromised. In this immunocompromised state, the HIV-infected individual is vulnerable to a variety of opportunistic viral, bacterial, fungal and parasitic infections. Opportunistic pathogens such as *Pneumocystis carinii*, *Cryptosporidium* and *Cryptococcus* seldom affect individuals with normally functioning immune systems but can be deadly in those infected with HIV. Patients who are severely immunocompromised are also at risk for the development of certain neoplasms, including Kaposi's sarcoma, human papillomavirus-related cervical cancers and some lymphomas. The development of opportunistic infections or neoplasms in a patient infected with HIV defines the acute immunodeficiency syndrome (AIDS). Patient who die of AIDS typically succumb to complications of an opportunistic infection or neoplasm.

Epidemiology of HIV infections

HIV has infected nearly 60 million people worldwide, and 40 million are presently living with the disease. The developing world accounts for 95% of infections, with over 25 million of those presently infected living in sub-Saharan Africa. The most important risk factor for acquiring HIV infection and succumbing to its complications is poverty.

Viral transmission occurs through direct contact with bodily fluids, most often semen or blood. Viral spread can occur via sexual contact, via parenteral exposure (intravenous drug abuse and transfusions) or via perinatal transmission. The latter can occur during pregnancy (transmission across the placenta), at delivery or during breastfeeding. Only 25% of children born to untreated HIV positive mothers will acquire the infection, although this rate can be decreased to less than 2% with aggressive antenatal and perinatal therapy. Over 70% of HIV infections occur via heterosexual transmission. HIV is more readily transmitted from the male to female than female to male.

Biology of HIV

HIV is a retrovirus. Its genetic material is carried as RNA wrapped in a viral protein coating. The viral surface expresses a receptor called gp120 that binds specifically to receptors on lymphoid cells. Binding promotes viral entry into host cells. Host receptors and co-receptors for viral entry include CCR5, a chemokine receptor on macrophages, CXCR4, a chemokine receptor expressed on T cells, and CD4, a marker for T helper cells that is also expressed on macrophages and dendritic cells. Once viral entry has occurred, infected cells will fuse with CD4+ T helper cells. Viral propagation will continue largely in CD4+ cells.

After entry into a host cell, the retrovirus uses reverse transcriptase to make a DNA copy of its viral RNA genome. The virus then uses an enzyme called integrase to insert its newly synthesized DNA into the host genome and the host cell machinery makes multiple copies of the HIV genome. The virus finally employs an enzyme called protease to reassemble the viral envelope. Viral particles then exit the host cell via budding to infect surrounding receptor laden immune cells. Multiple viral progeny will be produced within a single infected host cell before it expires.

Reverse transcriptase, integrase and protease are virus-specific enzymes. They can therefore serve as targets for directed therapeutic interventions. Nearly 20 medications are now available to treat HIV infections. None are curative and optimal therapies typically use combinations of 2–4 medications. Available antiretroviral medications inhibit two of the HIV-specific enzymes: the HIV protease (protease inhibitors) and the reverse transcriptase (RT) enzyme [nucleoside RT inhibitors (NRTI) and non-nucleoside RT inhibitors (NNRTI)]. Inhibitors of HIV viral entry are being developed.

In developed countries, careful therapeutic interventions, combined with close monitoring of CD4+ T cell counts and viral loads, have radically improved the prognosis for those infected with HIV. Further advances are challenged by the fact that the HIV reverse transcriptase enzyme makes many mistakes during replication of the viral genome. The virus has no way to readily correct these mistakes. This allows for rapid viral mutation and, unfortunately, the development of resistance to antiretroviral medications. In underdeveloped countries, where the prevalence of disease is highest, medications are scarce or completely unavailable.

Index

Numbers in roman denote index entry appears in text, *italics* in a figure and **bold** in a table